Elbow Arthritis

Guest Editors

JULIE E. ADAMS, MD
LEONID I. KATOLIK, MD

HAND CLINICS

www.hand.theclinics.com

May 2011 • Volume 27 • Number 2

SAUNDERS an imprint of ELSEVIER, Inc.

W.B. SAUNDERS COMPANY
A Division of Elsevier Inc.

1600 John F. Kennedy Blvd. ● Suite 1800 ● Philadelphia, Pennsylvania 19103

http://www.theclinics.com

HAND CLINICS Volume 27, Number 2
May 2011 ISSN 0749-0712, ISBN-13: 978-1-4557-0456-9

Editor: Debora Dellapena

Hand Clinics (ISSN 0749-0712) is published quarterly by Elsevier Inc., 360 Park Avenue South, New York, NY 10010-1710. Months of publication are February, May, August, and November. Business and Editorial Offices: 1600 John F. Kennedy Blvd., Ste. 1800, Philadelphia, PA 19103-2899. Customer Service Office: 3251 Riverport Lane, Maryland Heights, MO 63043. Periodicals postage paid at New York, NY and at additional mailing offices. Subscription price is $338.00 per year (domestic individuals), $540.00 per year (domestic institutions), $169.00 per year (domestic students/residents), $385.00 per year (Canadian individuals), $617.00 per year (Canadian institutions), $459.00 per year (international individuals), $617.00 per year (international institutions), and $223.00 per year (international and Canadian students/residents). Foreign air speed delivery is included in all *Clinics* subscription prices. All prices are subject to change without notice. **POSTMASTER:** Send address changes to *Hand Clinics*, Elsevier Health Sciences Division, Subscription Customer Service, 3251 Riverport Lane, Maryland Heights, MO 63043. Customer Service (orders, claims, online, change of address): Elsevier Health Sciences Division, Subscription Customer Service, 3251 Riverport Lane, Maryland Heights, MO 63043. Tel: 1-800-654-2452 (U.S. and Canada); 314-447-8871 (outside U.S. and Canada). Fax: 314-447-8029. E-mail: journalscustomerservice-usa@elsevier.com (for print support); journalsonlinesupport-usa@elsevier.com (for online support).

Reprints. For copies of 100 or more of articles in this publication, please contact the Commercial Reprints Department, Elsevier Inc., 360 Park Avenue South, New York, New York 10010-1710. Tel.: 212-633-3812; Fax: 212-462-1935; E-mail: reprints@elsevier.com.

Hand Clinics is covered in *MEDLINE/PubMed (Index Medicus), Current Contents/Clinical Medicine, EMBASE/Excerpta Medica,* and *ISI/BIOMED.*

Printed and bound by CPI Group (UK) Ltd, Croydon, CR0 4YY

Transferred to Digital Print 2011

Contributors

GUEST EDITORS

JULIE E. ADAMS, MD, MS
Assistant Professor of Orthopaedic Surgery, Department of Orthopaedic Surgery, University of Minnesota, Minneapolis, Minnesota

LEONID I. KATOLIK, MD, FAAOS
The Philadelphia Hand Center; Assistant Professor of Orthopaedic Surgery, Thomas Jefferson University, Philadelphia, Pennsylvania

AUTHORS

JULIE E. ADAMS, MD, MS
Assistant Professor of Orthopaedic Surgery, Department of Orthopaedic Surgery, University of Minnesota, Minneapolis, Minnesota

GEORGE S. ATHWAL, MD, FRCSC
Hand and Upper Limb Centre, St Joseph's Health Care, University of Western Ontario, London, Ontario, Canada

DARWIN D. CHEN, MD
Chief Resident, Department of Orthopaedic Surgery, Mount Sinai School of Medicine, New York, New York

MARK S. COHEN, MD
Professor; Director, Hand and Elbow Section; Director, Orthopaedic Education, Rush University Medical Center, Chicago, Illinois

LARRY D. FIELD, MD
Director, Upper Extremity Service, Mississippi Sports Medicine and Orthopaedic Center, Jackson, Mississippi

DAVID A. FORSH, MD
Chief Resident, Department of Orthopaedic Surgery, Mount Sinai School of Medicine, New York, New York

JEFFERY FRIEDRICH, MD
Associate Director, Combined Hand and Microvascular Surgery; Assistant Professor, Plastics and Reconstructive Surgery, Department of Surgery, University of Washington, Seattle, Washington

DOUGLAS P. HANEL, MD
Professor and Director, Combined Hand and Microvascular Surgery, Department of Orthopaedics and Sports Medicine, Harborview Medical Center, University of Washington, Seattle, Washington

MICHAEL R. HAUSMAN, MD
Robert K. Lippmann Professor of Orthopedic Surgery; Chief of Hand and Elbow Surgery, Department of Orthopaedic Surgery, Mount Sinai School of Medicine, New York, New York

LEONID I. KATOLIK, MD, FAAOS
The Philadelphia Hand Center; Assistant Professor of Orthopaedic Surgery, Thomas Jefferson University, Philadelphia, Pennsylvania

GRAHAM J.W. KING, MD, MSc, FRCSC
Professor, Division of Orthopaedic Surgery, Hand and Upper Limb Centre, University of Western Ontario, St Joseph's Health Care London, London, Ontario, Canada

ALEXANDRE LECLERC, MD, FRCSC,
Clinical Fellow, Division of Orthopaedic Surgery, Hand and Upper Limb Centre, St Joseph's Health Centre, London, Ontario, Canada

DONALD H. LEE, MD
Professor, Department of Orthopedic Surgery, Vanderbilt Orthopedic Institute, Vanderbilt University, Nashville, Tennessee

MICHAEL J. O'BRIEN, MD
Assistant Professor, Department of Orthopaedic Surgery, Tulane University School of Medicine, New Orleans, Louisiana

MARK T. REDING, MD
Associate Professor of Medicine, Division of Hematology, Oncology, and Transplantation, Center for Bleeding and Clotting Disorders, University of Minnesota, Minneapolis, Minnesota

LEE M. REICHEL, MD
Fellow, Combined Hand and Microvascular Surgery, University of Washington, Seattle, Washington; Assistant Professor, Department of Orthopedic Surgery, Baylor College of Medicine, Ben Taub General Hospital, Houston, Texas

FELIX H. SAVOIE III, MD
Lee C. Schlesinger Professor, Department of Orthopaedic Surgery; Director, Tulane Institute of Sports Medicine, Tulane University School of Medicine, New Orleans, Louisiana

SCOTT P. STEINMANN, MD
Professor, Department of Orthopedic Surgery, Mayo Clinic, Rochester, Minnesota

ALEXIS STUDER, MD
Instituto de Cirugía Plástica y de la Mano, Hospital Mutua Montañesa, Santander, Spain

BRETT P. WIATER, MD
Chief Resident, Department of Orthopaedics and Sports Medicine, University of Washington, Seattle, Washington

ROBERT W. WYSOCKI, MD
Assistant Professor, Department of Orthopaedic Surgery, Rush University Medical Center, Chicago, Illinois

Contents

Preface: Elbow Arthritis ix

Julie E. Adams and Leonid I. Katolik

Primary Osteoarthritis and Posttraumatic Arthritis of the Elbow 131

Robert W. Wysocki and Mark S. Cohen

Arthritis of the elbow resulting from either prior trauma or primary osteoarthritis is similar in that the end result is often a combination of pain and stiffness, but the location of the disorder can be different. Treatment decisions must be made on a case-by-case basis taking into account patient age, level of demand, and location and degree of degenerative changes. This article focuses primarily on the unique pathogenesis and general treatment rationale for primary osteoarthritis and post-traumatic arthritis of the elbow.

Rheumatoid Arthritis of the Elbow 139

Alexis Studer and George S. Athwal

Rheumatoid arthritis (RA) is the most common form of inflammatory arthropathy. RA is considered a disease of synovial joints, although it can cause various extra-articular manifestations. The synovium appears to be the primary target; however, investigations are ongoing to determine the exact etiology and pathoanatomy.

Hemophilic Arthropathy of the Elbow 151

Julie E. Adams and Mark T. Reding

Hemophilia is a hereditary disease in which circulating levels of coagulation factors are lacking, resulting in a propensity toward bleeding. Intra-articular hemorrhages are a hallmark of hemophilia and may lead a cascade of cytokine elaboration and inflammatory-mediated changes, which ultimately result in cartilage loss and arthropathy. Diarthrodial joints, such as the knee, elbow, and ankle, are most commonly affected. This article highlights issues surrounding hemophilic arthropathy of the elbow and focuses on preventive measures, management strategies of the hemophilic elbow, and treatment options for established arthropathy.

Osteocapsular Debridement for Elbow Arthritis 165

Leonid I. Katolik

Open capsular debridement is an excellent option for the treatment of elbow arthritis. This technique is particularly indicated in a patient population physiologically younger than 60 years. Given the young age and high functional demand of patients with primary osteoarthritis of the elbow, prosthetic replacement is generally not recommended. Open capsular debridement preserves the native joint and thus does not inherently require permanent activity modification as does replacement arthroplasty.

Arthroscopy for Arthritis of the Elbow 171

Felix H. Savoie III, Michael J. O'Brien, and Larry D. Field

Elbow arthroscopy has been used to treat patients with arthritis since the initial report of its efficacy by Savoie and colleagues in 1992. It has proved extremely useful as an adjunct treatment to decrease symptoms and increase function. A thorough knowledge of anatomy is essential for this modality to be used successfully. In young or active patients, it is the treatment of choice for arthritis of the elbow.

Arthrodesis of the Elbow   179

Lee M. Reichel, Brett P. Wiater, Jeffery Friedrich, and Douglas P. Hanel

Elbow arthrodesis (EA) is a procedure reserved for the salvage of failed elbow reconstruction or elbow injuries that defy reconstruction of a useful joint. Although arthrodesis of some joints is often straightforward and predictable, EA is technically difficult and associated with a high rate of complications. Furthermore, a successful EA does not translate to a gratifying clinical success. The functional limitations to activities of daily living and personal care are significant.

Elbow Interposition Arthroplasty   187

Darwin D. Chen, David A. Forsh, and Michael R. Hausman

End-stage elbow arthritis in young, active patients presents a challenging problem to the upper extremity surgeon. Total elbow arthroplasty is not a viable option in this population because of functional restrictions, limited implant survivorship, and the lack of an adequate salvage option. With the appropriate surgical indication, interposition arthroplasty can relieve severe pain, affording a functional elbow without severely proscribing permitted activities. In addition, bone stock is preserved, as are other reconstructive options for the future.

Linked Total Elbow Arthroplasty   199

Donald H. Lee

This article provides an overview of the current state of linked total elbow arthroplasty. Discussed are the general indications for using a linked implant and currently available implants. Disease-specific indications, contraindications, surgical technique, and rehabilitation are discussed. The overall results and disease-specific results, as well as complications after a linked elbow arthroplasty, are reviewed.

Unlinked and Convertible Total Elbow Arthroplasty   215

Alexandre Leclerc and Graham J.W. King

Total elbow arthroplasty (TEA) is still in its infancy if we compare it with other arthroplasties such as knee or hip. TEA designs have been evolving with experience; however, long-term outcome data remain limited. The designs of total elbow prostheses can be subdivided into 3 general categories: unlinked, linked, and convertible devices. This article focuses on unlinked and convertible prostheses.

Hemiarthroplasty of the Ulnohumeral and Radiocapitellar Joints   229

Scott P. Steinmann

Hemiarthroplasty involves replacement of the distal portion of the humerus without replacement of the ulna. This article reviews the literature on hemiarthroplasty of the ulnohumeral and radiocapitellar joints. It discusses the indications and outcomes of the technique and summarizes the author's experiences and results.

Index   233

Hand Clinics

FORTHCOMING ISSUES

August 2011

Hand Transplantation
W.P. Andrew Lee, MD, and
Gerald Brandacher, MD,
Guest Editors

November 2011

**New Advances in Wrist and
Small Joint Arthroscopy**
David J. Slutsky, MD,
Guest Editor

February 2012

Intrinsic Muscles of the Hand
Steven Green, MD, *Guest Editor*

May 2012

Elite Athlete's Hand and Wrist Injury
Michelle Carlson, MD, *Guest Editor*

RECENT ISSUES

November 2010

**Disorders of the Distal Radius Ulnar Joint
and Their Surgical Management**
Steven L. Moran, MD, and
Richard A. Berger, MD, PhD,
Guest Editors

August 2010

Technologic Advances and the Upper Extremity
Asif M. Ilyas, MD,
Guest Editor

May 2010

Complications in Hand Surgery
Jeffrey A. Greenberg, MD, MS,
Guest Editor

THE CLINICS ARE NOW AVAILABLE ONLINE!

Access your subscription at:
www.theclinics.com

Preface
Elbow Arthritis

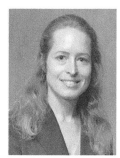 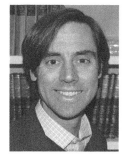

Julie E. Adams, MD, MS   Leonid I. Katolik, MD
Guest Editors

The elbow is essential as a stable platform to position the hand in space. Large stresses and forces transmitted through this joint make reconstruction and joint replacement challenging, while the unique anatomy of the joint adds to the complexity of surgical management. Arthritis of the elbow presents a problem in clinical practice and requires an understanding of the pathology present and the options available.

In this edition of *Hand Clinics*, evaluation and treatment of elbow arthritis will be explored. Disease-specific entities, including osteoarthritis, rheumatoid arthritis, and hemophilic arthropathy, will be explored by Drs Wysocki and Cohen, Drs Studer and Athwal, and Drs Adams and Reding. Various options for management will be presented including nonprosthetic options as well as joint replacement options. Open and arthroscopic debridement will be explored by Dr Katolik, and Drs Savoie, O'Brien, and Field. Indications and techniques for elbow fusion will be outlined by Drs Reichel, Wiater, Friedrich, and Hanel, while interposition arthroplasty will be explored by Drs Chen, Forsh, and Hausman. Joint replacement arthroplasty options will be reviewed, including constrained or semi-constrained implants discussed by Dr Lee, unconstrained implants by Drs Leclerc and King, and hemi-replacements by Dr Steinmann.

Recent interest and technology advancements in the evaluation and treatment options for elbow arthritis make this issue especially timely. It is our hope that this issue will prove useful in your practice.

Julie E. Adams, MD, MS
Department of Orthopaedic Surgery
University of Minnesota
2450 Riverside Avenue, R200
Minneapolis, MN 55454, USA

Leonid I. Katolik, MD
The Philadelphia Hand Center, P.C.
The Merion Building, Suite 200
700 South Henderson Road
King of Prussia, PA 19406, USA

E-mail addresses:
adams854@umn.edu (J.E. Adams)
likatolik@HANDCENTERS.com (L.I. Katolik)

Hand Clin 27 (2011) ix
doi:10.1016/j.hcl.2011.02.003
0749-0712/11/$ – see front matter

Primary Osteoarthritis and Posttraumatic Arthritis of the Elbow

Robert W. Wysocki, MD, Mark S. Cohen, MD*

KEYWORDS

- Primary osteoarthritis • Posttraumatic arthritis
- Elbow • Treatment

Arthritis of the elbow resulting from either prior trauma or primary osteoarthritis is similar in that the end result is often a combination of pain and stiffness, but the location of the disorder can be different. Treatment decisions must be made on a case-by-case basis taking into account patient age, level of demand, and location and degree of degenerative changes. This article focuses primarily on the unique pathogenesis and general treatment rationale for primary osteoarthritis and posttraumatic arthritis of the elbow.

BACKGROUND/PATHOGENESIS
Primary Osteoarthritis

Primary osteoarthritis of the elbow is uncommon and usually presents on the dominant side in middle-aged men who give a history of heavy use through sport or labor. Elbow osteoarthritis has a unique disease progression that provides a role for clinical success with debridement in its early stages, where such a procedure would traditionally be less successful in other joints such as the knee or hip.

The bony architecture of the ulnohumeral joint creates a high degree of articular congruity that leads to preservation of most the articular cartilage until the advanced stages of osteoarthritis. As a result, early disease typically presents with pain primarily at terminal extension and flexion associated with engaging osteophytes at the tips of the coronoid and olecranon, as well as their respective fossae (**Fig. 1**).[1–3] It is not until late-stage disease that there is pain throughout the arc of motion coinciding with diffuse articular degeneration. The impingement created by the engaging osteophytes not only causes pain, but, as they enlarge, the osteophytes become space-occupying lesions and lead to progressive stiffness resulting in secondary capsular contracture in time.

Primary osteoarthritis of the radiocapitellar joint alone is uncommon (**Fig. 2**). Patients presenting as such frequently have concomitant degenerative changes of the ulnohumeral joint. Therefore, before undertaking treatment of presumed isolated disease at the radiocapitellar joint, one must be certain that the patient's pain and tenderness is indeed located laterally, and that forearm rotation is typically more bothersome than elbow flexion and extension.

Rettig and colleagues[4] specifically studied morphologic characteristics in the osteoarthritic elbow compared with normal controls. No marked differences were seen. They found statistically significant increases in the ulnohumeral joint lateral facet angle on the anteroposterior radiograph as well as the deviation of the radiocapitellar line anteriorly from the center of the capitellum on the lateral radiograph. The investigators questioned the clinical significance of these findings, because the former was a difference of less than 5 degrees and the latter could be a manifestation of advanced elbow arthritis leading to anterior subluxation of the radius.

Posttraumatic Arthritis

Arthritis following elbow trauma can take several forms, usually dependant on the nature of the

Midwest Orthopaedics at Rush, 1611 West Harrison Street, Suite 400, Chicago, IL 60612, USA
* Corresponding author.
E-mail address: mcohen3@rush.edu

Hand Clin 27 (2011) 131–137
doi:10.1016/j.hcl.2011.02.001

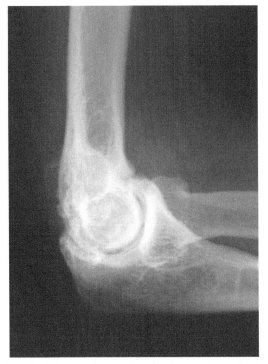

Fig. 1. Lateral radiograph of elbow osteoarthritis demonstrating impinging osteophytes in the anterior and posterior ulnohumeral joints as well as on the anterior radial head.

original trauma. One of the more common sources is radiocapitellar arthritis after malunion of a displaced intra-articular radial head fracture (see **Fig. 2**). In such cases, similar to cases of symptomatic radiocapitellar osteoarthritis, patients usually present with laterally based elbow pain that localizes well to the radiocapitellar joint and pain with forearm rotation more than elbow flexion and extension. Arthritis secondary to malunion of

intra-articular distal humerus fracture or proximal ulna fracture can be found as well.

In addition to identifying the arthritic area of the elbow in such patients, it is equally important to assess whether there was any elbow instability at the time of injury in the form of a fracture dislocation, and whether there are signs or symptoms of ongoing instability. The presence of ongoing instability limits the operative options for management in favor of arthroplasty or arthrodesis.

EVALUATION
History

When taking a history from a patient with posttraumatic or primary arthritis of the elbow, there are several important factors to address. It is critical to identify the current complaint. If the primary complaint is pain, one should attempt to localize it (ie, radiocapitellar joint, ulnohumeral joint) and confirm whether the patient has pain only at the extremes of flexion and extension or whether there is pain throughout the arc of motion. If stiffness is the primary complaint, it is important to assess whether the patient primarily lacks flexion, extension, or both, and whether there is any significant dysfunction secondary to the condition or whether it is simply an asymmetry the patient has noticed. Patient selection is also critical in elbow stiffness operations, given the extensive rehabilitation required and potential for limited clinical success in the noncompliant or uninformed patient.

The expectations and demand level of the patient must also be considered, because this greatly influences the treatment options, especially for advanced disease when considering arthroplasty alternatives. Special consideration must be given in the case of the previously operated elbow with posttraumatic arthritis. Any history or concerns for

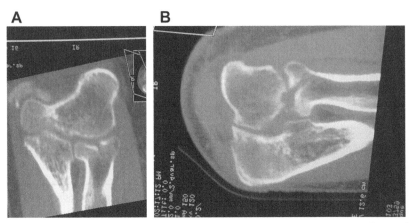

Fig. 2. (A) Anteroposterior and (B) lateral radiographs of radiocapitellar post-traumatic arthritis after radial head fracture.

prior or ongoing infection must be carefully elicited, especially if bony nonunion is present, because arthroplasty options may be contraindicated in this setting. If infection is at all suspected, serologic markers for infection should be obtained and an aspiration of the elbow joint performed, with the aspirate analyzed for cell count and Gram stain. All attempts should made to obtain previous operative reports and records. The history should also routinely include specific questioning regarding any neurologic symptoms, because disorders of especially the ulnar nerve are common with elbow arthritis regardless of the cause.

Physical Examination

Inspection- should include documentation of previous surgical incisions and any areas of poor soft tissue coverage or contracture that would affect further operative intervention. Bilateral range of motion of both the elbow and forearm should be documented and it should be noted where within that range of motion pain is reproduced. One must be cautious in evaluating the radiocapitellar joint in cases of primary osteoarthritis, because it frequently seems degenerated but is not usually a pain generator unless there is significant preoperative pain with forearm rotation.[5–7] Elbow stability is critical to assess in the posttraumatic setting. This assessment can be done by looking for frank instability or, more commonly, apprehension with provocative tests such as the posterolateral drawer, or by obtaining stress radiographs. Special attention should be paid to a thorough neurologic examination, in particular of the ulnar nerve, because it commonly shows signs of compression, which the patient may not recognize as such. There should be a low threshold for obtaining electrodiagnostic studies if neurologic function is in question.

Imaging

All attempts should also be made to obtain and review previous radiographs in the posttraumatic or previously operated patient. A full set of current radiographs is obtained. Although rheumatoid arthritis frequently shows symmetric joint-space narrowing, the osteoarthritic elbow often shows preservation of the joint space centrally with degenerative changes and osteophytosis anteriorly and posteriorly (see **Fig. 1**). The congruency of the ulnohumeral and radiocapitellar joints should be confirmed. The degree of joint-space narrowing and osteophyte formation for the ulnohumeral and radiocapitellar joints should be considered separately and any evidence of fracture malunion should be identified. Any factors that would be contributing to motion loss should also be identified, including not only impinging osteophytes but also heterotopic ossification in the posttraumatic setting.

Rettig and colleagues[4] devised a classification system for radiographic staging of elbow osteoarthritis, and showed that the effectiveness of debridement diminishes as stage of disease increases. Class I elbows show marginal osteophyte formation at the ulnohumeral joint but no arthritic changes of the radiocapitellar joint. Class II elbows have progressed to include degenerative changes of the radiocapitellar joint, and class III elbows also have subluxation of the radiocapitellar joint.

Computed tomography (CT), often combined with intra-articular contrast injection, is helpful in primary osteoarthritis in identifying loose bodies, defining the borders of heterotopic ossification, and identifying osteophytes poorly seen on plain radiographs such as shelf osteophytes in the olecranon fossa, coronoid fossa, and radial fossa, posterior capitellar osteophytes, and osteophytes in the medial gutter adjacent to the ulnar nerve (**Fig. 3**). CT is also useful in posttraumatic arthritis not only for the reasons listed earlier but also to evaluate for suspected fracture nonunion and better characterize deformity. Magnetic resonance imaging (MRI) and bone scintigraphy are primarily only used in cases of suspected infection.

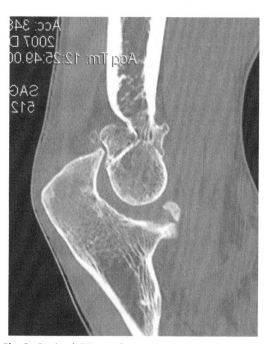

Fig. 3. Sagittal CT scan demonstrating complex osteophytes in the anterior and posterior ulnohumeral joints.

TREATMENT PRINCIPLES

Both osteoarthritis and posttraumatic arthritis are treated conservatively in the early stages. Nonsteroidal antiinflammatory medications and activity modification are encouraged, but adherence to the latter is often difficult for the laborer or athlete. The role of viscosupplementation for elbow arthritis was studied by van Braken and Eygendaal,[8] who found minimal decrease in pain and activity impairment at 3 months, but no lasting benefits at 6 months in 18 patients. There were no complications from the injections.

When conservative treatment has failed, regardless of whether the arthritis has resulted from osteoarthritis or trauma, there are several factors to consider in planning surgical intervention. The first factor is the patient's primary complaint. Patients with primary complaints of stiffness rather than pain in the setting of mild or moderate arthritis are ideal candidates for open or arthroscopic debridement and capsular release. The same can usually be applied to patients with primary osteoarthritis and pain just at the extremes of motion, because they usually present with painful engaging osteophytes anteriorly and/or posteriorly but with much of the articular surface well preserved. Patients with diffuse joint-space narrowing and pain throughout the arc of motion suggestive of more advanced disease are not good candidates for debridement and are more likely to benefit from procedures such as distraction interposition arthroplasty, total elbow arthroplasty, or elbow arthrodesis.

Regardless of whether open or arthroscopic debridement is chosen, the treatment principles in these cases are the same. Loss of flexion and anterior impingement symptoms are addressed by resection of anterior bony impingement, often between the coronoid and cornoid fossa but occasionally the radial head and radial fossa, and release or excision of the posterior capsule as needed. Conversely, loss of extension and posterior impingement are addressed by resection of posterior bony impingement between the olecranon and olecranon fossa and release or excision of the anterior capsule as needed.

The early description of open debridement for elbow osteoarthritis, also known as the Outerbridge-Kashiwagi procedure,[9] was through a posterior approach that allowed direct visualization for debridement of the posterior ulnohumeral joint, followed by debridement of the coronoid through a circular cavity in the humerus just proximal to the trochlea (**Fig. 4**). Although providing excellent exposure posteriorly, this procedure makes access to the radiocapitellar joint and the

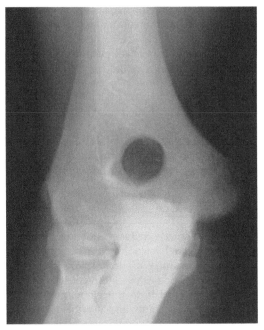

Fig. 4. Anteroposterior radiograph after the Outerbridge-Kashiwagi procedure showing the circular defect above the trochlea.

anterior capsule difficult and thus has limited indications. Open debridement is now more commonly performed using medial and/or lateral exposures that provide full access to the structures of the anterior and posterior elbow. Several series of open debridement have shown improvements in pain as well as increases in range of motion averaging 20 to 30 degrees.[10–12]

Advances in elbow arthroscopy have established a role in treating many cases of primary osteoarthritis arthroscopically, especially in young patients. Excellent results with improvements in pain and range of motion have been reported.[13,14] The indications for both open and arthroscopic debridement include those listed earlier, but the authors believe there are cases in which open treatment is superior, including elbows with significant heterotopic ossification in which the tissue planes are difficult to establish arthroscopically, cases with significant deformity, and most elbows that have been previously operated on, especially if the ulnar nerve has been transposed or the radial head was exposed. If the radial head has been affected in this way, potential scarring of the radial nerve to the anterior capsule should be suspected. Open ulnar nerve decompression and/or transposition should be considered along with open or arthroscopic elbow debridement if the patient has signs (a positive Tinel test) or symptoms of ulnar neuropathy preoperatively or if the patient

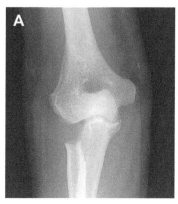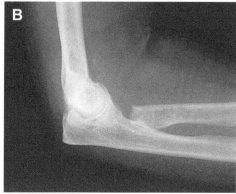

Fig. 5. (A) Anteroposterior and (B) lateral radiographs after radial head excision.

cannot flex past 100 to 110 degrees before surgery, because the increased postoperative flexion would put the nerve at risk of traction neuropathy.[10] The specific indications, techniques, and results of open and arthroscopic debridement for elbow arthritis are discussed by Leonid I. Katolik; and Savoie and colleagues respectively elsewhere in this issue.

Isolated radiocapitellar arthritis exists as a separate entity, most commonly a posttraumatic disorder after radial head fracture but occasionally as primary osteoarthritis. These patients often present with more limitation of elbow flexion and extension than pronation and supination but do have painful forearm rotation. Pain with rotation most commonly differentiates the patient with symptomatic radiocapitellar arthritis from the patient with painful ulnohumeral arthrosis and incidental asymptomatic radiocapitellar disease. For the former, when no instability is present, good results for increased motion and decreased pain have been reported for both open[15] and arthroscopic[5,6] radial head resection (**Fig. 5**). The latter frequently does well with treatment of the ulnohumeral arthritis but not the radiocapitellar

joint despite a degenerative appearance arthroscopically, thus avoiding the risk of increased load across the ulnohumeral joint after radial head excision.[7]

Radial head arthroplasty (**Fig. 6**) is another treatment option in this patient population, with proposed benefits compared with radial head excision that include prevention of proximal migration of the radius and prevention of ulnohumeral arthritis from repeated valgus load. Arthroplasty is especially useful in the posttraumatic setting with instability, but does carry a risk of degenerative changes of the capitellum in time. Resurfacing of the capitellum in this setting has been described but has not been studied in depth.[16,17] The indications, preferred implant designs, and outcomes of radial head arthroplasty continue to be refined as midterm outcome studies become available.

Advanced degenerative disease involving most of the ulnohumeral joint is typically not amenable to successful treatment by debridement alone. For the younger patient with inflammatory arthritis (<30–40 years old) or posttraumatic/osteoarthritis (<60 years old), interposition arthroplasty or elbow arthrodesis are the primary surgical options

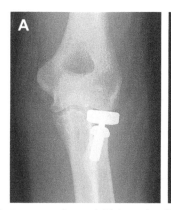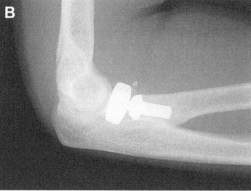

Fig. 6. (A) Anteroposterior and (B) lateral radiographs after metallic radial head arthroplasty.

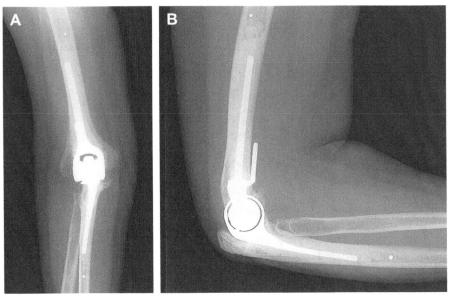

Fig. 7. (*A*) Anteroposterior and (*B*) lateral radiogrpahs after total elbow arthroplasty.

because they have increased durability in the higher-demand patient and do not carry the same lifting restriction as total elbow arthroplasty (2.3–4.5 kg). Although good results for interposition arthroplasty with Achilles allograft have been reported,[18] there is a significant risk for elbow instability after surgery, making well-preserved bone stock essential for a good outcome.[18,19] Total elbow arthroplasty is best indicated for the low-demand patient with inflammatory arthritis, or the older patient (>60 years old) with posttraumatic arthritis or osteoarthritis who is willing to comply with the substantial postoperative restrictions placed on the arm following total elbow arthroplasty (**Fig. 7**). Specific attention is paid to interposition and linked/unlinked total elbow arthroplasty discussed by Donald H. Lee; and Leclerc and colleagues respectively elsewhere in this issue.

SUMMARY

Treatment of posttraumatic arthritis and osteoarthritis of the elbow must be individualized on a case-by-case basis depending on location of disease, age/demand level of the patient, and stage of disease. Early stage disease is most amenable to debridement. The indications for open versus arthroscopic debridement continue to be refined, but early results of both seem to show similar effectiveness. Both procedures can be performed safely, but arthroscopic debridement requires advanced skill in elbow arthroscopy. Later-stage disease typically requires reconstructive procedures, with the specific choice of

treatment based largely on patient age and demand level. The indications, techniques, and results for each of the treatments described earlier are discussed elsewhere in this edition.

REFERENCES

1. Cheung EV, Adams R, Morrey BF. Primary osteoarthritis of the elbow: current treatment options. J Am Acad Orthop Surg 2008;16:77–87.
2. Gallo RA, Payatakes A, Sotereanos DG. Surgical options for the arthritic elbow. J Hand Surg Am 2008;33:746–59.
3. Kokkalis ZT, Schmidt CC, Sotereanos DG. Elbow arthritis: current concepts. J Hand Surg Am 2009; 34:761–8.
4. Rettig LA, Hastings H 2nd, Feinberg JR. Primary osteoarthritis of the elbow: lack of radiographic evidence for morphologic predisposition, results of operative debridement at intermediate follow-up, and basis for a new radiographic classification system. J Shoulder Elbow Surg 2008;17:97–105.
5. McLaughlin RE 2nd, Savoie FH 3rd, Field LD, et al. Arthroscopic treatment of the arthritic elbow due to primary radiocapitellar arthritis. Arthroscopy 2006; 22:63–9.
6. Menth-Chiari WA, Ruch DS, Poehling GG. Arthroscopic excision of the radial head: clinical outcome in 12 patients with post-traumatic arthritis after fracture of the radial head or rheumatoid arthritis. Arthroscopy 2001;17:918–23.
7. Kelly EW, Bryce R, Coghlan J, et al. Arthroscopic debridement without radial head excision of the osteoarthritic elbow. Arthroscopy 2007;23:151–6.

8. van Brakel RW, Eygendaal D. Intra-articular injection of hyaluronic acid is not effective for the treatment of post-traumatic osteoarthritis of the elbow. Arthroscopy 2006;22:1199–203.

9. Kashiwagi D. Osteoarthritis of the elbow joint: intra-articular changes and the special operative procedure; Outerbridge-Kashiwagi method (O-K method). In: Kashiwagi D, editor. The elbow joint. Philadelphia: Elsevier; 1985. p. 177–88.

10. Antuna SA, Morrey BF, Adams RA, et al. Ulnohumeral arthroplasty for primary degenerative arthritis of the elbow: long-term outcome and complications. J Bone Joint Surg Am 2002;84:2168–73.

11. Morrey BF. Primary degenerative arthritis of the elbow. Treatment by ulnohumeral arthroplasty. J Bone Joint Surg Br 1992;74:409–13.

12. Phillips NJ, Ali A, Stanley D. Treatment of primary degenerative arthritis of the elbow by ulnohumeral arthroplasty. A long-term follow-up. J Bone Joint Surg Br 2003;85:347–50.

13. Krishnan SG, Harkins DC, Pennington SD, et al. Arthroscopic ulnohumeral arthroplasty for degenerative arthritis of the elbow in patients under fifty years of age. J Shoulder Elbow Surg 2007;16:443–8.

14. Adams JE, Wolff LH 3rd, Merten SM, et al. Osteoarthritis of the elbow: results of arthroscopic osteophyte resection and capsulectomy. J Shoulder Elbow Surg 2008;17:126–31.

15. Broberg MA, Morrey BF. Results of delayed excision of the radial head after fracture. J Bone Joint Surg Am 1986;68:669–74.

16. Heijink A, Morrey BF, Cooney WP 3rd. Radiocapitellar hemiarthroplasty for radiocapitellar arthritis: a report of three cases. J Shoulder Elbow Surg 2008;17:e12–e15.

17. Tomaino MM. The emerging role for Uni-Elbow arthroplasty. Am J Orthop (Belle Mead NJ) 2008;37:26–8.

18. Larson AN, Morrey BF. Interposition arthroplasty with an Achilles tendon allograft as a salvage procedure for the elbow. J Bone Joint Surg Am 2008;90:2714–23.

19. Nolla J, Ring D, Lozano-Calderon S, et al. Interposition arthroplasty of the elbow with hinged external fixation for post-traumatic arthritis. J Shoulder Elbow Surg 2008;17:459–64.

Rheumatoid Arthritis of the Elbow

Alexis Studer, MD[a], George S. Athwal, MD, FRCSC[b],*

KEYWORDS

- Rheumatoid arthritis • Elbow • Synovectomy
- Interpositional arthroplasty • Elbow arthroplasty
- Arthroscopy

Rheumatoid arthritis (RA) is the most common form of inflammatory arthropathy, affecting between 0.5% and 1% of the general population, with twice as many women as men affected.[1] RA is considered a disease of synovial joints, although it can cause various extra-articular manifestations. The synovium appears to be the primary target; however, investigations are ongoing to determine the exact etiology and pathoanatomy. Genetic predisposition, with the presence of the HLA-DR4 gene, involvement of activated immune cells, clonal expansion of the cells in pathologic lesions, and the response to immunosuppressive therapy would suggest that the disease is immune mediated.[2]

CLINICAL FEATURES

The clinical manifestations of RA can be variable; however, characteristic features include an insidious onset of morning stiffness, usually lasting more than 30 minutes, together with a symmetric polyarthritis involving mainly metacarpophalangeal (MCP) and proximal interphalangeal joints (PIP) of the hand. Typically, larger joints become symptomatic as the disease progresses. Atypical presentations, such as an asymmetric pattern of joint involvement or pronounced systemic complaints, can make the diagnosis challenging. The diagnosis of RA is primarily clinical, although blood tests may reveal the presence of autoantibodies to immunoglobulin G (IgG). The American College of Rheumatology, in association with the

European League Against Rheumatism, has developed a classification system focusing on the early features of the disease, therefore emphasizing prompt diagnosis and rapid initiation of effective treatments. This new classification system is based on confirmed synovitis in at least 1 joint that cannot be better explained by alternative diagnosis and obtaining a total score of 6 or greater in 4 domains (**Table 1**).[3]

Early in the disease course, the most frequently affected joints are the MCP, PIP, and wrist. Involvement of the elbow joint is also common at a frequency that varies from 20% to 65%. Lehtinen and colleagues[4,5] found that 61% of patients diagnosed with RA had radiological evidence of elbow involvement. Isolated presentation of RA of the elbow, however, occurs in only about 5% of the patients.

The earliest pathologic abnormality in RA is acute synovitis, which will spontaneously resolve in about 10% of patients. The synovium becomes hypertrophied and congested, which increases intra-articular pressure, leading to capsular distension causing elbow pain and contracture. The fact that patients may hold the elbow in a flexed position to minimize pain may itself worsen the flexion contracture. One of the earliest findings on clinical examination is this loss of elbow extension, together with posterolateral boggy swelling. Additional clinical manifestations can include nodules, bursitis and antecubital synovial cysts, which can compress adjacent nerves. Radiographically, soft tissue edema and periarticular osteoporosis can

[a] Instituto de cirugía plástica y de la mano, Hospital Mutua Montañesa, C/Calderon de la Barca 16. Entlo Izq, 39002 Santander, Spain
[b] Hand and Upper Limb Centre, St Joseph's Health Care, University of Western Ontario, 268 Grosvenor Street, London, ON, Canada N6A 4L6
* Corresponding author.
E-mail address: gsathwal@hotmail.com

Hand Clin 27 (2011) 139–150
doi:10.1016/j.hcl.2011.01.001

Table 1
The 2010 American College of Rheumatology classification criteria for rheumatoid arthritis

	Score
Who should be tested?	
1. Patients who have at least 1 joint with definite clinical swelling and synovitis not better explained by another disease	
Classification criteria (score ≥6/10 is needed for classification)	
A. Joint involvement	
1 large joint	0
2–10 large joints	1
1–3 small joints (with or without a large joint)	2
4–10 small joints (with or without a large joint)	3
>10 joints (at least 1 small joint)	5
B. Serology (at least 1 positive test is needed)	
Negative RF and ACPA	0
Low-positive RF and ACPA	2
High positive RF and ACPA	3
C. Acute-phase reactants (at least 1 test positive test is needed)	
Normal CRP and ESR	0
Abnormal CRP and ESR	1
D. Duration of symptoms	
<6 weeks	0
≥6 weeks	1

Abbreviations: ACPA, anticitrullinated protein antibody; CRP, C-reactive protein; ESR, erythrocyte sedimentation rate; RF, rheumatoid factor.

Data from Aletaha D, Neogi T, Silman AJ, et al. 2010 Rheumatoid arthritis classification criteria. An American College of Rheumatology/European League against rheumatism collaborative initiative. Arthritis Rheum 2010;62(9):2569–81.

be seen early (Larsen grade 1). As the disease progresses, proliferative granulation tissue or pannus starts to attack the joint at its margins where it is not protected by cartilage. In radiographic terms, this stage is represented by joint space narrowing and periarticular bony erosions (Larsen stage 2). At later stages, the inflammatory pannus projects into the joint and extends across the joint, producing cartilage and bone damage. The loss of articular cartilage is typically diffuse and symmetric within the joint when compared with osteoarthritis, where the joint space narrowing is more focal or asymmetric. The radiographic features of this stage are bony erosion and the formation of subchondral cysts (Larsen stage 3). In the final stages of disease, the erosive pannus extends into tendons and ligaments predisposing to instability. Clinically, painful clicking or snapping may be present. As the disease progresses, patients can experience deformity, subluxation, dislocation, fracture, fragmentation, and bone loss (Larsen stage 4). With continuing synovial inflammation and cartilage damage, the articular cavity may become infiltrated with fibrous tissue that may ossify with resultant ankylosis (Larsen grade 5).[6]

Rheumatoid nodules can frequently be found around the elbow area and are more common in seropositive disease, which precludes a more severe erosive pattern. Nodules are usually asymptomatic, but can ulcerate and become infected. When planning to excise a nodule as part of another procedure, such as an elbow arthroplasty, the surgeon must take great care in protecting the soft tissues, as the skin is often thin and fragile.

IMAGING

Standard anteroposterior and lateral radiographs are sufficient to characterize the extent of disease progression. As mentioned in the preceding section, the Larson classification grades joint involvement based on osteopenia, joint space narrowing, erosions, and articular damage.[7] This general classification scheme is divided into 4 grades with the recent addition of a fifth grade by Connor and Morrey (**Fig. 1**, **Table 2**).[8] Advanced imaging, in the form of computed tomography or

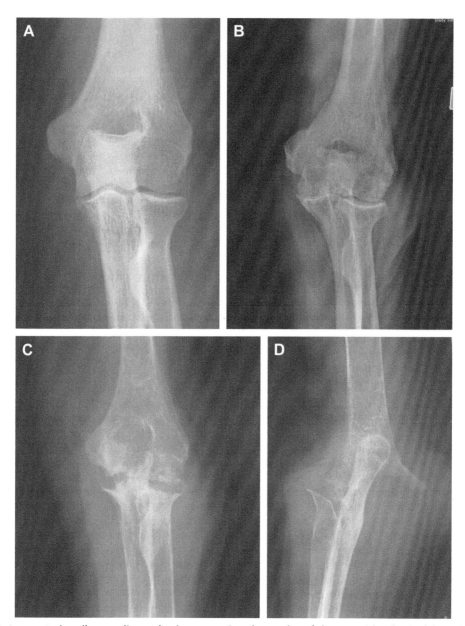

Fig. 1. Anteroposterior elbow radiographs demonstrating the grades of rheumatoid arthritis. (*A*) Grade 1 osteoporosis. (*B*) Grade 2 articular narrowing. (*C*) Grade 3 architectural changes of the bones. (*D*) Grade 4 gross destruction of the joint.

magnetic resonance imaging, is used as the disease progresses to assist with the determination of indications for surgery.

TREATMENT

There is no cure for RA, and the goals of treatment are to decrease pain, reduce inflammation, delay disease progression, and to maintain long-term function of the joint. The ideal treatment strategy for RA is not yet known. Fortunately, recent advances in medical management have had a major impact on controlling disease progression.

Activity modification has been shown to be beneficial for patients with RA; however, rest without physiotherapy can lead to joint stiffness and muscle atrophy. Therefore, the proper balance between rest and physical activity is important. Formal occupational and physical therapy can educate patients on joint protection by avoiding forces that are damaging and by maintaining motion and strength.

Table 2
Clinic classification of the rheumatoid elbow

Grade	Description
1	No radiographic changes. Slight abnormality: periarticular osteopenia with accompanying soft-tissue swelling; mild-to-moderate synovitis
2	Minimal or no architectural distortion. Mild-to-moderate joint space narrowing
3	Architectural alteration, such as thinning of the olecranon, or resorption of the trochlea or capitellum; variable reduction in joint space with or without cyst formation
4	Severe articular damage; gross destruction and instability
5	Ankylosis; absence of an identifiable ulnohumeral joint on the anteroposterior and lateral radiographs (mature osseous trabeculation crossing the ulnohumeral joint)[8]

Data from Larsen A, Dale K, Eek M. Radiographic evaluation of rheumatoid arthritis and related conditions by standard reference films. Acta Radiol Diagn 1977;18:481–91.

Disease modifying antirheumatic drugs (DMARDs) such as methotrexate, sulfasalazine, and hydroxychloroquine are used as the basis for medical treatment. Recently tumor necrosis factor (TNF) inhibitors, such as etanercept, infliximab, and adalimumab have been developed and shown to be effective in controlling disease progression. Combination therapy, the use of more than one medication concurrently, has gained favor. The combination of different DMARDs[9] or the combination of a TNF-α inhibitor with methotrexate[10] has proven to be more effective than a single form of treatment. Additionally, combination therapy with DMARDs has been shown to provide the added benefit without increasing toxicity. Recent studies suggest that starting DMARD therapy earlier may improve long-term outcomes. Recently, a meta-analysis reported sustained suppression of the rate of radiologic disease progression after 5 years with early DMARD therapy.[11] An interval of time may exist in which the introduction of DMARD therapy can result in a change in the natural course of the disease. Although the use of DMARDs and TNF inhibitors has proven to be very effective in controlling disease progression and decreasing the rate of surgical treatment, they have not yet managed to

achieve remission, the ultimate long-term goal of medical therapy.

Intra-articular elbow steroid injections can be effective for the short-term relief of acute inflammatory exacerbations. The repeated use of intra-articular steroids, however, may not be desirable because of the detrimental effects of steroids on articular cartilage.

When nonoperative therapies fail and pain becomes unmanageable, surgery is offered. Other important indications for operative management are the loss of range of motion, instability, or pathologic fractures. Surgical options are synovectomy, interposition arthroplasty, and total elbow replacement. Other surgical options include arthrodesis and resection arthroplasty, which tend to be poorly tolerated.

PREOPERATIVE CARE

All patients with RA should be evaluated, monitored, and medically optimized by a rheumatologist before surgical intervention. When considering surgery on patients with RA, the surgeon should be familiar with several perioperative factors unique to RA.

Cervical spine stability must be assessed before surgery. In patients with RA, it is not uncommon to have cervical spine instability, with the atlantoaxial pattern being the most common type. Cervical instability can be identified by history, physical examination, and imaging. Standard radiographs should include anteroposterior, lateral, openmouth odontoid, and flexion/extension lateral views. The anterior atlantodens interval (ADI: distance between the posterior edge of the ring of C1 and the anterior edge of the odontoid) should be assessed, and instability is present if there is a greater than 3.5 mm difference between flexion and extension radiographs. The posterior atlantodens interval (PADI: distance between the posterior aspect of the odontoid to the anterior surface of the posterior C1 ring) also should be measured and a minimum threshold value of 14 mm is required. The PADI has been shown to be a more useful prognosticator in RA patients than the ADI.

Many patients with RA receive medications that can increase the risk of wound healing problems and infection. Glucocorticoids over a prolonged period of time and in high doses (>40 mg/d) increase the risk of wound healing problems and adrenal axis suppression.[12] Recent studies suggest that low doses of methotrexate (2–8 mg weekly) do not increase the risk of infection and that continuing drug treatment during the perioperative period can suppress disease flares, especially in severe disease.[13,14] The current trend is to continue methotrexate unless certain risk factors are present (elderly patients, renal impairment, diabetes, lung or liver disease, alcohol abuse, or >10 mg/d of prednisone usage), in which case it is advisable to withhold for the week before and after surgery.[15] Regarding the remaining antirheumatic drugs in current use, the available data cannot support any clear evidence-based recommendations on perioperative use or discontinuation. The data on the perioperative usage of anti-TNF agents are unclear.[16,17] Most recent reports advise discontinuing the medication for a minimum of 4 weeks preoperatively, and restarting it 2 weeks after surgery.[18] Aspirin and cyclooxygenase inhibitors also should be withheld for at least 7 to 10 days before surgery to decrease the risk of perioperative bleeding.

SURGICAL OPTIONS
Synovectomy

Synovectomy has been advocated for early treatment of RA in patients with uncontrolled synovitis despite receiving 6 months of medical treatment. Patients with early grades of arthritis, Larsen 2 or 2, are the best candidates for synovectomy. Generally, synovectomy procedures have better results in patients with some preservation of joint space with minimal bony deformity. Nevertheless, younger patients or patients with a pauciarticular disease may be candidates, despite having advanced disease and bony destruction, due to the limited surgical options available for this patient group. Synovectomy can be performed surgically or chemically. Surgical synovectomy can be performed either open or arthroscopically (**Fig. 2**). The primary goal of synovectomy is pain relief through the reduction of synovial tissue and fluid, and therefore intra-articular pressure.

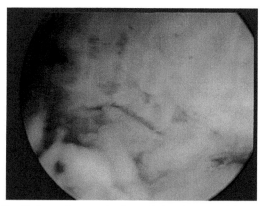

Fig. 2. An arthroscopic view of the rheumatoid pannus before synovectomy.

Postoperatively, synovectomy outcomes are better maintained with a lower incidence of recurrence if patients continue to be treated with DMARDs.

Chemical synovectomy or synoviorthesis (destruction of synovial tissue using intra-articular injection of radioactive or chemical substances) has been used in an attempt to eradicate the synovium of rheumatoid and hemophilic patients. Unfortunately, the use of radioactive (32P chromic phosphate,[19] yttrium-90[20] or rhenium-186[21]) or chemical substances (osmic acid,[22] oxitetracycline clorhydrate) has a success rate of less than 50%.[20,21] The elbow and knee joints responded significantly better than shoulders and ankles, although one should be aware of the subcutaneous location of these joints and the increased risk of soft tissue problems.[23,24] Studies suggesting the potential for cartilage necrosis and possible induction of malignancy have limited the use of these agents.[25] Synoviorthesis, however, is an alternative to surgical synovectomy in chronic synovitis that fails to respond to conservative treatment, especially in patients who are not candidates for surgery.

Open synovectomy, with or without radial head excision, is an established treatment option for patients with RA of the elbow.[20–23,25–33] The procedure may be conducted under a regional or general anesthetic. A posterior midline incision or a direct lateral incision can be used. The deep lateral approach involves an extensile Kocher approach with preservation of the lateral collateral ligament. The radial head is examined and retained if minimally symptomatic with preserved forearm rotation. In cases where pain and symptoms are related to the radial head with restricted forearm range of motion, radial head excision is indicated. Rymaszewski and colleagues[34] recommended replacing the radial head with an implant to limit changes in elbow kinematics and load transfer. In contrast, other investigators have reported good results with radial head excision.[30,35] However, in patients with medial collateral ligament insufficiency, radial head resection without replacement is contraindicated due to potential instability. In cases where the medial side of the elbow joint is heavy involved with synovitis that cannot be adequately addressed from the lateral side, a medial approach is warranted. The literature, however, has shown no clinically significant differences between single lateral or two-incision synovectomies.[35]

Fuerst and colleagues[29] evaluated the long-term results and survival rate (no further operations) in 85 patients treated with open synovectomy. They concluded that early synovectomy (Larsen 1/2) had a better survival rate at 10 years that synovectomy performed at advanced disease stages. Gendi and colleagues[30] observed that result deteriorates with time. After the first year, the cumulative survival rate declined gradually by an average of 2.6% per year. The overall failure rate of synovectomy was 46% during an average follow-up period of 6.5 years. They observed a higher chance of success when forearm rotation was reduced to below 50% without significant limitation of flexion–extension. In general, open synovectomy has a 71% to 93% satisfactory rate at short- to intermediate-term follow-up.[36] Unfortunately as mentioned previously, these results tend to deteriorate over time, dropping to a 50% satisfactory outcome at longer-term follow-up.

The most common complication after open synovectomy is recurrence. The rate of recurrent synovitis after open synovectomy ranges from 16% to 43%.[27,31,35] The reoperation rate in this patient cohort can be as high as 25% with longer-term follow-up.[36] Repeated synovectomy can be recommended; however, the outcomes are less predictable. Other more successful alternatives, such as total elbow replacement, should be considered; however, there is some literature reporting higher a higher total elbow arthroplasty (TEA) complication rate after a failed synovectomy.[37] Stiffness and instability are less common, although the frequency increases during the more advanced stages of the disease. Nerve injury is rare after open synovectomy.

Arthroscopic synovectomy is becoming increasingly popular, despite being a technically demanding procedure with a risk of neurologic complications. Several factors make arthroscopic synovectomy an attractive alternative to open synovectomy, such as the ability to conduct the surgery on an out-patient bases, improved visualization of the entire joint, better postoperative pain control, a lower risk of infection, smaller incisions with a lower likelihood of wound problems, and the perceived ability to participate in earlier and more active rehabilitation. Arthroscopic synovectomy, however, is more challenging than other arthroscopic procedures for several reasons. Visualization is impaired by the abundant synovitis; the capsular volume is decreased. reducing the space for the surgeon to operate, and finally, the capsule is generally thinner. All of these factors increase the risk of neurovascular injury. The relative contraindications to arthroscopic synovectomy are advanced disease, altered bony and soft tissue anatomy, a poor soft tissue envelope, and surgeon inexperience.

The procedure is typically performed under general anesthesia with tourniquet control.

Arthroscopic synovectomy of the elbow is divided into 3 parts: anterior, posterior, and posterior radiocapitellar compartments. Within each compartment, synovectomy and debridement are done with great care taken to protect the neurologic structures with safe technique and liberal use of arthroscopic retractors.

There are no high level-of-evidence clinical trials that compare open with arthroscopic synovectomy in patients with RA. Articles published suggest that better results can be expected when dealing with less affected elbows but that regardless of the joint condition, outcomes will deteriorate over time. In 1997, Lee and Morrey[38] reported that the results of arthroscopic synovectomy deteriorate more rapidly than after open synovectomy, concluding that it was mainly because of the limitations of the arthroscopic technique. In 2002, Horiuchi and colleagues[39] reported on 20 patients after subtotal arthroscopic synovectomy (no medial gutter synovectomy), with the results indicating good-to-excellent outcomes in 71% at 2 years. At final follow-up (8 years), however, only 43% of the elbows were graded as good to excellent, with 5 recurrences (24%) of synovitis. They concluded that arthroscopic synovectomy is a reliable procedure to alleviate pain, especially in early stages of disease. Tanaka and colleagues[40] also reported better results in early stages. They also found that outcomes were better in those patients with a preoperative flexion arc greater than 90°.

The complications of arthroscopic synovectomy are similar to open techniques, with recurrence of synovitis being the most frequent. In the case of failure, repeated synovectomy can be performed, although less predictable results should be anticipated. The infection rate is reported to range between 0.8% and 2%. A complication specific to arthroscopy is the development of synovial fistulae, which can be avoided by suturing closed the arthroscopy portals. One of the most devastating complications of elbow arthroscopy is nerve injury. In one series investigating risks of nerve injury following arthroscopy of the elbow, the most significant risk factors for the development of a temporary nerve palsy were an underlying diagnosis of RA and presence of a contracture.[41] This risk may be lowered by careful attention to safe technique, avoidance of cases with altered anatomy, and the use of retractors.

Distraction/Interposition Arthroplasty

Interposition arthroplasty is a salvage procedure that consists of interposing fascia, dermis, or Achilles tendon allograft between the humerus and ulna. The ideal patient is a younger patient with incapacitating arthritis, mostly limited to the elbow, who is not a candidate for arthroplasty. This operation does not fully eliminate pain, nor allow the patient to regain a full arc of motion, but it is considered a safe intermediate-term procedure that preserves bone stock for future prosthetic alternatives. The use of this procedure in RA is limited due to often multiple joint involvement. RA patients typically place lower demands on their joints and are candidates for alternative, more reliable procedures such as replacement arthroplasty. RA patients also often present with poor bone stock, poor bone quality, and some degree of instability, which precludes an optimum result. An active infection is an absolute contraindication, and gross elbow instability with bone loss is a relative contraindication.

To date, the optimal resection of bone, the ideal choice of interposition material, the role of ligament repairs/reconstruction, and the use of a distraction device have not been fully determined. When conducting the procedure, a minimum amount of bone should be resected to maintain overall joint shape and to minimize bone resorption. Preservation of native anatomy, including the radial head, will assist with maximizing joint stability. The medial and lateral collateral ligaments should be preserved, repaired, or reconstructed, as stability is a prerequisite for a good outcome.

The goals of interposition arthroplasty are to relieve pain and provide a functional range of motion. The outcomes of interposition arthroplasty are not as good as total elbow arthroplasty; however, significant pain relief can be expected in 60% to 70% of well-selected patients. Cheng and Morrey[42] studied 13 patients (10 post-traumatic and 3 inflammatory) who underwent interpositional arthroplasty at a mean follow-up of 63 months. Eight patients (62%) had an excellent or good result by the objective criteria of the Mayo elbow performance score, and 4 patients went on to total elbow arthroplasty because of pain and instability. The patient numbers were low; however, the success rate was similar when performed for RA or post-traumatic disease. Larson and Morrey,[43] in their study of 45 patients (34 post-traumatic patients and 11 inflammatory patients), treated with Achilles tendon allograft found a significant association between poorer outcome and preoperative instability and suggested that instability on physical examination and pain without elbow dysfunction should be considered as contraindications to interposition arthroplasty.

The complications of interpositional arthroplasty include instability, stiffness, heterotopic bone formation, infection, bone resorption, incomplete pain relief, and triceps rupture.

Total Elbow Arthroplasty

The advanced stages of RA are best treated with total elbow arthroplasty. Prior to 1970, end-stage elbow RA was treated with resection arthroplasty, interposition arthroplasty, or arthrodesis. Over the last 40 years, advances in implant technology and surgical techniques have made total elbow replacement a reliable procedure. Presently, the success rate of elbow arthroplasty in patients with RA approaches the results of hip and knee replacements.[44] In younger patients, however, the revision rate of total elbow arthroplasty is higher. Celli and Morrey[45] published a 22% revision rate at 91 months in patients younger than 40 years of age. Nonreplacement options such as synovectomy and interposition arthroplasty are still preferable in this group when possible.

Total elbow arthroplasty is absolutely contraindicated in patients with active infection. Patients who are good candidates for an alternative surgical procedure or who are unwilling to comply with arthroplasty activity and weight restrictions should not be treated with total elbow replacement. Previous infection is a strong relative contraindication. However, recent studies suggest that total elbow arthroplasty can be successfully performed in selected patients using a staged debridement with negative cultures.[46]

Total elbow arthroplasty implants are classified as linked, unlinked, or convertible. A decision to use an unlinked or linked device depends on bone loss, the status of the capsuloligamentous tissues, the surgeon's experience. and the expected demands of the patient.

Linked implants such as the Coonrad-Morrey (Zimmer, Warsaw, IN, USA), GSB-III (Gschwend-Scheier-Bahler, Zimmer, Warsaw, IN, USA) (Allopro) and the Discovery (Biomet, Parsippany, NJ, USA) all incorporate a sloppy hinge. This loose hinge replicates more accurately the semiconstrained biomechanics of the native elbow, allowing 6° to 10° of varus–valgus motion. Linked devices have broader indications than unlinked implants, as they are suitable in the setting of gross deformity, instability with deficient ligaments, or extensive humeral or ulnar bone loss (**Fig. 3**).

Unlinked implants do not have a linkage and rely on the inherent stability provided by the implant configuration, the dynamic effects of the elbow musculature, and the capsuloligamentous structures. The most popular designs are the Souter-Strathclyde (Stryker Howmedica Osteonics, London, UK), Kudo (Biomet, Warsaw, IN, USA),

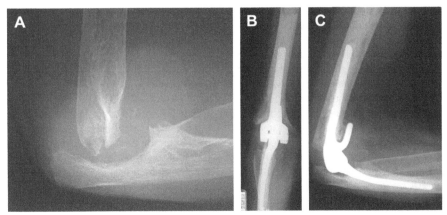

Fig. 3. Anteroposterior (see **Fig. 1**D) and lateral radiographs (*A*) of a 75-year-old woman with longstanding rheumatoid arthritis with elbow involvement consisting of ulnar and humeral bone loss. Total elbow arthroplasty with a linked semiconstrained implant provided pain relief, stability, and a functional range of motion (*B, C*).

Capitello-condylar (Johnson & Johnson, Warsaw, IN, USA), Sorbie-Questor (Wright Medical Technologies, Arlington, TN, USA) and Pritchard ERS (Depuy, Warsaw, IN, USA). The concept in these implants is that load is shared between the ligaments, capsule, and muscles; therefore, decreased forces are experienced by the implants and polyethylene articulation. This is theorized to lead to decreased loosening and failure, but this theory has yet to be confirmed in clinical studies.

Convertible devices allow the versatility of selecting a linked or unlinked articulation intraoperatively, depending on patients' characteristics (**Fig. 4**).[47] Convertible implants also allow conversion from an unlinked to a linked device if late instability develops. The Latitude (Tornier Incorporated, Stafford, TX, USA) and Acclaim (DePuy) prostheses are examples of convertible implants.[48] The Latitude device can also be inserted as a hemiarthroplasty and converted, if required, to linked or unlinked total elbow prosthesis without revision of the humeral stem.

Total elbow arthroplasty is typically conducted under a general anesthetic. There are several

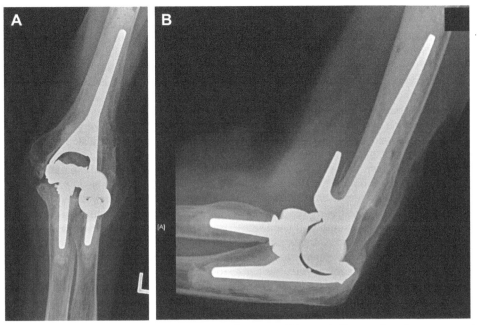

Fig. 4. Anteroposterior and lateral radiographs (*A, B*) of a convertible total elbow arthroplasty system placed in to a patient with rheumatoid arthritis in the unlinked configuration. (*Courtesy of* Dr Graham King, MD.)

described surgical approaches for elbow arthroplasty; however, the selected approach typically depends on the surgeon's experiences and preferences. There are two general classifications of approaches, the triceps reflecting/dividing and the triceps-on approaches. Some examples of the triceps reflecting/dividing approaches are the Bryan-Morrey,[49] the triceps splitting,[50] the extended Kocher,[51] and the triceps reflecting anconeus pedicle (TRAP) approaches.[52] The advantage of the triceps reflecting/dividing approaches is that they offer better visualization of the joint, however, at the expense of complications such as extensor weakness and triceps repair dehiscence. A commonly used triceps-on approach is the paratricipital approach,[53,54] which exposes the joint from medial and lateral arthrotomies. The advantage of the triceps-on approaches is maintenance of the extensor mechanism, which will not require postoperative protection.

Postoperative rehabilitation protocols vary depending on the type of triceps approach used (triceps reflecting vs triceps-on) and the style of implant (linked vs unlinked). No rigid guidelines exist for postoperative patient restrictions; however, the authors recommend that patients avoid lifting more than 1 kg repetitively or more than 4 kg as a single event.

The outcomes of total elbow arthroplasty for RA are generally good. Pain relief, joint stability, and a functional arc of motion can be achieved in over 90% of patients. In 1998, Gill and Morrey[44] reported the Mayo Clinic's experience with the Coonrad-Morrey (linked semiconstrained) implant in 78 patients. The Kaplan Meier curve for the Coonrad-Morrey prosthesis revealed a survivorship of 94% at 12 years follow-up, which is similar to that of knee and hip replacement. Eleven serious complications were recorded (14%), with only 2 cases of infection and 4 cases of aseptic loosening. In another series, Hildebrand and colleagues[55] compared the results of TEA in patients with inflammatory arthritis versus traumatic or post-traumatic conditions using the Coonrad-Morrey prosthesis. The authors found no significant difference in range of motion; however, patients with inflammatory arthritis reported better functional outcomes.

The reported outcomes of unlinked arthroplasty are variable. In 1993, Ewald and colleagues[56] reported good results in 202 unlinked capitellocondylar arthroplasties with a 1.5% incidence of postoperative dislocation and 1.5% incidence of aseptic loosening. The experience reported by other investigators with the same prosthesis was less favorable, with an instability rate of up to 20% in some studies.[57,58] Van Der Lugt and colleagues[59] reported a 10-year survival rate of 77% in 204 patients with the Souter-Strathclyde implant. The authors reported dislocation in 2% of patients and aseptic loosening in 12% of patients at 6.4 years follow-up.

There are no prospective randomized trials comparing the outcomes of different TEA systems.[60] Little and colleagues[61] compared the outcomes of three different implants (Coonrad-Morrey, Kudo, Souter-Strathclyde) in a prospective consecutive cohort of patients. The three implants provided similar pain relief and range of motion; however, the 5-year survival rate of the Souter-Strathclyde was lower than the Kudo and Coonrad-Morrey. The authors concluded that a linked prosthesis (Coonrad-Morrey) prevented dislocation, without increasing the rate of aseptic loosening.

At present, there is only one study reporting the outcomes of a convertible device. Bassi and colleagues[48] published the results of 36 Acclaim prostheses, reporting marked pain relief and an improvement in movement and function. At 36 months follow-up, the authors reported that the early results of this implant are encouraging. Complications included 11 patients experiencing an intraoperative condyle fracture and 2 patients developing implant instability that required conversion to a linked prosthesis.

The complication rate continues to be higher in total elbow arthroplasty than in other large joint replacements such as the hip and knee. The global percentage of complications that require revision surgery or have permanent consequences is approximately 28 plus or minus 13%.[62] The most common complication continues to be aseptic loosening, although the most serious is infection.

Early complications include wound healing problems and ulnar nerve symptoms. Ulnar nerve paresthesias can be found in over 25% of patients with a total elbow replacement; fortunately, most are transient. Aseptic loosening is the most frequent late complication that leads to the highest number of revisions.

Infection rates in TEA remain higher than in other joint replacements, with reported rates ranging from 1% to 11%. In addition, eradication of elbow infection is more difficult than in other joint replacements. Risk factors for infection are immunosuppression, diabetes mellitus, poor nutrition, obesity, multiple prior surgeries, and prolonged wound drainage. The increasing use of disease-remitting agents in RA is an area of potential concern because of the increased rate of infection.

Other complications after TEA include stiffness, heterotopic ossification, periprosthetic fractures, and triceps insufficiency. Celli and colleagues[63] reported 2% of patients having surgery to correct triceps weakness after total elbow replacement.

Other options for patients with RA that are rarely indicated are resection arthroplasty and arthrodesis. Resection arthroplasty is most frequently indicated for infections that are difficult to eradicate. Arthrodesis also has very few indications. Fusion of the elbow in any position is poorly tolerated, especially in rheumatoid patients with polyarticular disease who are unable to compensate for a fused elbow due to limited mobility of adjacent joints.

SUMMARY

Although RA is typically a disease of the small joints, it can affect the elbow in greater than 50% of patients. In recent years, there have been encouraging advances in the medical management of RA. Improved medical management strategies have led to improved disease control and a decreased frequency of surgery. The use of targeted biologic therapy, the administration of combination therapy, and earlier initiation of disease-modifying therapy are on the rise as further data emerge regarding their efficacy, utility, and safety. When surgery is needed in the early stages of disease, there is a trend toward arthroscopic synovectomy. In the later stages, total elbow arthroplasty remains the best option to decrease pain and to improve function and range of motion.

REFERENCES

1. Clayton ML. Historical perspectives on surgery of rheumatoid hand. Hand Clin 1989;5(2):111–4.
2. Genovese MC, Harris ED Jr. Treatment of rheumatoid arthritis. In: Harris ED, Budd RC, Firestein GS, et al, editors. Kelly's textbook of rheumatology. 7th edition. Philadelphia (PA): Saunders; 2004. p. 1079–99.
3. Aletaha D, Neogi T, Silman AJ, et al. 2010 Rheumatoid arthritis classification criteria. An American College of Rheumatology/European League against rheumatism collaborative initiative. Arthritis Rheum 2010;62(9):2569–81.
4. Lehtinen JT, Kaarela K, Kauppi MJ, et al. Bone destruction patterns of the rheumatoid elbow: a radiographic assessment of 148 elbows at 15 years. J Shoulder Elbow Surg 2002;11(3):253–8.
5. Lehtinen J, Kaarela K, Ikavalko M, et al. Incidence of elbow involvement in rheumatoid arthritis. A 15-year endpoint study. J Rheumatol 2001;28(1):70–4.
6. Resnick D. Rheumatoid arthritis and the seronegtive spondyloarthropathies: radiographic and pathologic concepts. In: Resnick DL, Kransdorf MJ, editors. Bone and joint imaging. 3rd edition. Philadelphia (PA): Elsevier, Saunders; 2002. p. 837–90.
7. Larsen A, Dale K, Eek M. Radiographic evaluation of rheumatoid arthritis and related conditions by standard reference films. Acta Radiol Diagn 1977;18: 481–91.
8. Connor PM, Morrey BF. Total elbow arthroplasty in patients who have juvenile rheumatoid arthritis. J Bone Joint Surg Am 1998;80(5):678–88.
9. O'Dell JR, Haire CE, Erikson N, et al. Treatment of rheumatoid arthritis with methotrexate alone, sulfasalazine and hydroxychloroquine, or a combination of all three medications. N Engl J Med 1996;334:1287–91.
10. Maini R, St Clair EW, Breedveld F, et al. Infliximab (chimeric antitumor necrosis factor alpha monoclonal antibody) versus placebo in rheumatoid arthritis patients receiving concominant methotrexate: a randomized phase III trial. ATTRACT Study Group. Lancet 1999;354(9194):1932–9.
11. Finckh A, Liang MH, van Herckenrode CM, et al. Long-term impact of early treatment on radiographic progression in rheumatoid arthritis: a meta-analysis. Arthritis Rheum 2006;55(6):864–72.
12. Anstead GM. Steroids, retinoids, and wound healing. Adv Wound Care 1998;11(6):277–85.
13. Worthing AB, Cupps TR. The rheumatic cause of elbow instability. Hand Clin 2008;24(1):79–80.
14. Murata K, Yasuda T, Ito H, et al. Lack of increase in postoperative complication with low-dose methotrexate therapy in patients with rheumatoid arthritis undergoing elective orthopedic surgery. Mod Rheumatol 2006;16(1):14–9.
15. Rosandich PA, Kelley 3rd JT, Conn DL. Perioperative management of patients with rheumatoid arthritis in the era of biologic response modifiers. Curr Opin Rheumatol 2004;16(3):192–8.
16. Wendling D, Balblanc J-C, Brousse A, et al. Surgery in patients receiving antitumour necrosis factor alpha treatment in rheumatoid arthritis: an observational study on 50 surgical procedures. Ann Rheum Dis 2005;64:1378–9.
17. den Broeder AA, Creemers MC, Fransen J, et al. Risk factors for surgical site infections and other complications in elective surgery in patients with rheumatoid arthritis with special attention for antitumor necrosis factor: a large retrospective study. J Rheumatol 2007;34(4):689–95.
18. Dixon WB, Lunt M, Watson KD, et al. Anti-TNF therapy and the risk of serious postoperative infection: results from the BSR biologics register (BSRBR). Ann Rheum Dis 2007;66(Suppl 2):118.
19. Rivard GE, Girard M, Belanger R, et al. Synoviorthesis with colloidal 32P Chromic phosphate for the treatment of hemophilic arthropathy. J Bone Joint Surg Am 1994;76(4):482–8.
20. Stucki G, Bozzone P, Treuer E, et al. Efficacy and safety of radiation synovectomy with yttrium-90. Retrospective long-term analysis of 164 applications in 82 patients. Br J Rheumatol 1993;32(5):383–6.

21. Gobel D, Gratz S, von Rothkirch T, et al. Radiosynoviorthesis with rhenium-186 in rheumatoid arthritis: a prospective study of three treatment regimens. Rheumatol Int 1997;17(3):105–8.

22. Oka M, Rekonen A, Ruotsi A. The fate and distribution of intra-articularly injected osmium tetroxide (Os-191). Acta Rheumatol Scand 1969;15(1):35–42.

23. Mitchel N, Laurin C, Shepard N. The effect of osmium tetroxide and nitrogen mustard on normal articular cartilage. J Bone Joint Surg Br 1973;55(4):814–21.

24. Bickels J, Isaakov J, Kollender Y, et al. Unacceptable complications following intra-articular injection of Yttrium 90 in the ankle joint for diffuse pigmented villonodular synovytis. J Bone Joint Surg Am 2008; 90(2):326–8.

25. Lipton JH, Messner HA. Chronic myeloid leukemia in a woman with Still's disease treated with 198Au synoviorthesis. J Rheumatol 1991;18(5):734–5.

26. Brumfield RH Jr, Resnick CT. Synovectomy of the elbow in rheumatoid arthritis. J Bone Joint Surg Am 1985;67(1):16–20.

27. Copeland SA, Taylor JG. Synovectomy of the elbow in rheumatoid arthritis. J Bone Joint Surg Br 1979; 61(1):69–73.

28. Ferlic DC, Patchett CE, Clayton ML, et al. Elbow synovectomy in rheumatoid arthritis: long-term results. Clin Orthop 1987;220:119–25.

29. Fuerst M, Fink B, Rüther WJ. Survival analysis and longterm results of elbow synovectomy in rheumatoid arthritis. J Rheumatol 2006;33(5):892–6.

30. Gendi NS, Axon JM, Carr AJ, et al. Synovectomy of the elbow and radial head excision in rheumatoid arthritis. Predictive factors and long-term outcome. J Bone Joint Surg Br 1997;79(6):918–23.

31. Inglis AE, Ranawat CS, Straub LR. Synovectomy and debridement of the elbow in rheumatoid arthritis. J Bone Joint Surg Am 1971;53(4):652–62.

32. Mäenpää HM, Kuusela PP, Kaarela K, et al. Reoperation rate after elbow synovectomy in rheumatoid arthritis. J Shoulder Elbow Surg 2003;12(5):480–3.

33. Smith SR, Pinder IM, Ang SC. Elbow synovectomy in rheumatoid arthritis: present role and value of repeat synovectomy. J Orthop Rheumatol 1993;6:155–7.

34. Rymaszewski LA, Mackay I, Amis AA, et al. Long-term effects of excision of the radial head in rheumatoid arthritis. J Bone Joint Surg Br 1984;66(1):109–13.

35. Porter BB, Richardson C, Vainio K. Rheumatoid arthritis of the elbow: the results of synovectomy. J Bone Joint Surg Br 1974;56(3):427–37.

36. Cil A, Morrey BF. Synovecomy of the elbow. In: Morrey BF, Sanchez-Sotelo J, editors. The elbow and its disorders. 4th edition. Philadelphia (PA): Saunders Elsevier; 2009. p. 921–34.

37. Whaley A, Morre BF, Adams R. Total elbow arthroplasty after previous resection of the radial head and synovectomy. J Bone Joint Surg Am 2005; 87(1):47–53.

38. Lee BP, Morrey BF. Arthroscopic synovectomy of the elbow for rheumatoid arthritis. A prospective study. J Bone Joint Surg Br 1997;79(5):770–2.

39. Horiuchi K, Momohara S, Tomatsu T, et al. Arthroscopic synovectomy of the elbow in rheumatoid arthritis. J Bone Joint Surg Am 2002;84(3):342–7.

40. Tanaka N, Sakahashi H, Hirose K, et al. Arthroscopic and open synovectomy of the elbow in rheumatoid arthritis. J Bone Joint Surg Am 2006;88(3):521–5.

41. Kelly EW, Morrey BF, O'Driscoll SW. Complications of elbow arthroscopy. J Bone Joint Surg Am 2001; 83(1):25–34.

42. Cheng SL, Morrey BF. Treatment of the mobile, painful arthritic elbow by distraction interposition arthroplasty. J Bone Joint Surg Br 2000;82(2):233–8.

43. Larson AN, Morrey BF. Interposition arthroplasty with an Achilles tendon allograft as a salvage procedure for the elbow. J Bone Joint Surg Am 2008;90(12): 2714–23.

44. Gill DR, Morrey BF. The Coonrad-Morrey total elbow arthroplasty in patients who have rheumatoid arthritis. A ten- to fifteen-year follow-up study. J Bone Joint Surg Am 1998;80(9):1327–35.

45. Celli A, Morrey BF. Total elbow arthroplasty in patients forty years of age or less. J Bone Joint Surg Am 2009;91(6):1414–8.

46. Yamaguchi K, Adams RA, Morrey BF. Semiconstrained total elbow arthroplasty in the context of treated previous infection. J Shoulder Elbow Surg 1999;8(5):461–5.

47. Gramstad GD, King GJ, O'Driscoll SW, et al. Elbow arthroplasty using a convertible implant. Tech Hand Up Extrem Surg 2005;9(3):153–63.

48. Bassi RS, Simmons D, Ali F, et al. Early results of the acclaim elbow replacement. J Bone Joint Surg Br 2007;89(4):486–9.

49. Bryan RS, Morrey BF. Extensive posterior exposure of the elbow: a triceps sparing approach. Clin Orthop 1982;166:188–92.

50. Azar FM, Wright PE. Arthroplasty of the shoulder and elbow. In: Canale ST, editor. Campbell's Operative Orthopedics, vol. 1. 9th edition. Mosby St Louis; 1998. p. 505–13.

51. Kocher T. Textbook of operative surgery. 3rd edition. London: A. and C. Black; 1911.

52. O'Driscoll SW. The triceps-reflecting anconeus pedicle (TRAP) approach for distal humeral fractures and nonunions. Orthop Clin North Am 2000; 31(1):91–101.

53. AlonsoLlames M. Bilaterotricipital approach to the elbow. Its application in the osteosynthesis of supracondylar fractures of the humerus in children. Acta Orthop Scand 1972;42(6):479–90.

54. Boorman RS, Page WT, Weldon EJ, et al. A triceps-on approach to semiconstrained total elbow arthroplasty. Tech Shoulder Elbow Surg 2003;4(3): 139–44.

55. Hildebrand KA, Patterson SD, Regan WD, et al. Functional outcome of semiconstrained total elbow arthroplasty. J Bone Joint Surg Am 2000;82(10): 1379–86.

56. Ewald FC, Simmons ED, Sullivan JA, et al. Capitello-condylar total elbow replacement in rheumatoid arthritis. Long-term results. J Bone Joint Surg Am 1993;75(4):498–507.

57. Weiland AJ, Weiss AP, Willis RP, et al. Capitellocon-dylar total elbow replacement. A long-term follow-up study. J Bone Joint Surg Am 1989;71(2):217–22.

58. King GJ, Adams RA, Morrey BF. Total elbow arthro-plasty: revision with use of a noncustom semicon-strained prosthesis. J Bone Joint Surg Am 1997; 79(3):394–400.

59. van der Lugt JC, Geskus RB, Rozing PM. Primary Souter-Strathclyde total elbow prosthesis in rheumatoid arthritis. J Bone Joint Surg Am 2004; 86(3):465–73.

60. Little CP, Graham AJ, Carr AJ. Total elbow arthro-plasty: a systematic review of the literature in the English language until the end of 2003. J Bone Joint Surg Br 2005;87(4):437–44.

61. Little CP, Graham AJ, Karatzas G, et al. Outcomes of total elbow arthroplasty for rheumatoid artritis: comparative study of three implants. J Bone Joint Surg Am 2005;87(11):2349–448.

62. Morrey BF, Voloshin I. Complication of elbow replae-ment arthroplasty. In: Morrey BF, Sanchez-Sotelo J, editors. The elbow and its disorders. 4th edition. Phila-delphia (PA): Saunders Elsevier; 2009. p. 849–61.

63. Celli A, Arash A, Adams R, et al. Triceps insuffi-ciency following total elbow arthroplasty. J Bone Joint Surg Am 2005;87(9):1957–64.

Hemophilic Arthropathy of the Elbow

Julie E. Adams, MD, MS[a],*, Mark T. Reding, MD[b]

KEYWORDS

- Hemophilia • Elbow arthritis • Hemophilic arthropathy
- Elbow arthropathy

Hemophilia A and B result from an X-linked deficiency or deficit of factor VIII or factor IX, respectively, which leads to a propensity toward bleeding.[1–3] Severity of disease is classified by the level of the circulating clotting factor; levels greater than 5%, 1% to 5%, and less than 1% correspond to mild, moderate, and severe hemophilia, respectively.[1,2,4] There are roughly 18,000 persons with hemophilia in the United States, approximately 60% of whom are severely affected. Patients with mild disease typically experience bleeding complications only after major trauma or surgery, whereas those with moderate disease have bleeding after minor trauma and may occasionally have spontaneous bleeds.[1] In severe cases, spontaneous intra-articular bleeds are common and may involve the knee, elbow, or ankle, or other joints.[1,4] Diarthrodial hinged joints, such as the knee, elbow, and ankle, may be more vulnerable to hemarthrosis because of their relatively larger synovial content when compared with shoulder or hip joints and are indeed the most commonly affected joints in hemophilia.[1,3–5] Recurrent intra-articular hemorrhage may lead to hemophilic arthropathy, which causes significant morbidity in the hemophilia population.[2–5] Because of the elbow's role in positioning the hand in space, involvement of the elbow joint can be particularly problematic for these patients.

In the acute setting of a hemarthrosis, the joint is swollen, painful, and warm, with decreased range of motion. Typically in this setting, the joint responds adequately to factor replacement and rest, returning to normal over the course of days to weeks. Appropriate treatment, therefore, is brief immobilization, factor replacement, and gradual return to activity.[6,7]

Subacute arthropathy ensues after a critical threshold of synovitis develops after repeated hemarthroses; the joints become boggy with synovial hyperplasia and effusion. Synovial hyperplasia results in more bleeds and worsening joint deterioration.

At the chronic stage, bony changes develop with microcysts, cartilage loss from lack of support for the articular surface, and enzymatic changes from the synovium. Ligamentous and capsular changes also eventually develop.[6,7]

The pathophysiology of hemophilic arthropathy begins with recurrent intra-articular bleeds.[3,8,9] Although it is generally thought that there is a correlation between recurrent bleeds and arthropathy, little is known about the process and the sufficient number of bleeds that may result in what seems to be an irreversible joint destruction process.[1,8,10] In vitro experiments suggest that exposure to a concentration of 10% of the maximum joint capacity for more than 2 days is required to result

Financial Disclosure/Relationships/Conflict of Interest: The authors have nothing to disclose and no conflict relevant to the subject matter in the article.
Funding: NA. No funding was received.
[a] Department of Orthopaedic Surgery, University of Minnesota, 2450 Riverside Avenue, R200, Minneapolis, MN 55454, USA
[b] Division of Hematology, Oncology, and Transplantation, Center for Bleeding and Clotting Disorders, University of Minnesota, Mayo Mail Code 420, 420 Delaware Street SE, Minneapolis, MN 55455, USA
* Corresponding author.
E-mail address: adams854@umn.edu

Hand Clin 27 (2011) 151–163
doi:10.1016/j.hcl.2011.01.007
0749-0712/11/$ – see front matter © 2011 Elsevier Inc. All rights reserved.

in irreversible changes; however, the in vivo implications remain less clear.[11]

The causative process of hemophilic arthropathy seems to occur along at least 2 independent but related pathways. Firstly, an inflammatory synovial component exists in response to intra-articular bleeds.[9] In a murine model, intra-articular bleeds result in elevated synovial levels of the cytokines IL-1β, IL-6, KC and MCP-1.[12] The elaboration of these inflammatory mediators has a deleterious effect on the cartilage.[9] Cytokines activate monocytes and macrophages to produce hydrogen peroxide, which, in the presence of hemosiderin and iron, can result in the synthesis of hydroxyl radicals.[9,13] After recurrent bleeds, hemosiderin deposits are consumed by macrophages, and a hypertrophic synovium develops with increased vascularity and an inflammatory infiltration and vascularity. This hypertrophic synovium also has a deleterious effect on the cartilage because lysosomal enzymes are released from the synovium, which result in articular cartilage destruction.[3,14,15]

Moreover, independent of synovial-based inflammation, it seems that the presence of hematoma in the joint also directly and independently interferes with cartilage metabolism, resulting in inhibition of proteoglycan and aggrecan synthesis and cartilage destruction by way of increased catabolism of these components, with a final common pathway of hemophilic arthropathy.[3,9,14,15] In vitro and canine models suggest that there is an impairment of cartilage matrix synthesis and enhanced matrix degradation after hemarthrosis; this effect persists up to 10 weeks, well beyond the period by which hematoma is absorbed and resolved.[9,13,16–18] Chondrocyte apoptosis seems to be a primary mechanism of impaired cartilage matrix synthesis.[19,20] Eventually, the hypertrophic synovium becomes fibrotic and scarred. The joint cartilage is destroyed, and the joint becomes contracted and arthritic.[3] In addition, in patients who are skeletally immature, the synovium and increased vascular supply can result in gross abnormalities and angular deformities that persist into adulthood (**Fig. 1**).[3,8]

CLINICAL FEATURES OF HEMOPHILIC ARTHROPATHY OF THE ELBOW

Although joint involvement in hemophilia in the knee and ankle has been well studied, there is limited information regarding the elbow. The elbow is the third most commonly affected joint but lags greatly behind the knee and ankle. In 1 series, the elbow joint was the most common site of joint discomfort in only 7% of patients, whereas the ankle was bothersome in about 45% of patients.[21] Although it may be a less common site of pain, hemophilic arthropathy involving the elbow can have serious functional consequences, and the elbow is the most common site of involvement in hemophilic arthropathy of the upper extremity.[4,22,23]

There are discrepancies among series about whether the dominant or nondominant elbow is most commonly affected, and about half of patients have bilateral involvement.[4,8,22,24]

Children with hemophilia rarely experience bleeding in the absence of trauma or surgery during the first year of life, and hemarthroses begin typically after a child begins to walk.[25] Pettersson and colleagues[26] demonstrated that radiographic joint changes were rare before the age of 3 years, whereas after age of 6 years, almost all untreated severe hemophiliacs develop some radiographic changes.

Longitudinal studies suggest elbow involvement can be problematic after 5 years of age.[8] In one series,[27] 42% of all bleeding episodes in these patients occurred in the upper extremities, and the rate of bleeding was greatest in those patients aged between 23 and 30 years. Pain was not a prominent feature in this patient subset as more than 75% of the elbows were pain free. Most commonly, clinical findings included diminished motion, chronic synovitis, and muscle wasting. Typically pronation is the first motion to be lost, although extension may be affected to a greater extent in hemophilic arthrosis.[4,25,27] Gamble and colleagues[27] investigated long-term effects of recurrent hemarthroses on elbow and wrist motion in patients with hemophilia. Pronation was the first motion to be lost in these patients. When patients were compared by 1 of 3 age groups (<15, 15–25, and >25 years), supination was decreased by about 35% in the oldest group of patients compared with the youngest group. Although flexion decreased by an average of 25°, loss of elbow extension was the largest difference. Patients in the older than 25 years group averaged a 34° loss of extension for the dominant elbow, and loss of elbow flexion and extension were also greater for dominant versus nondominant extremities.

It has been suggested that concomitant lower extremity involvement may make elbow joint arthropathy either more common or more symptomatic because of the need for gait aids to support body weight using the arms. In one series, only 1 patient had elbow involvement without concomitant lower extremity joint involvement and all other patients had concomitant knee involvement. In addition, unilateral elbow joint involvement was observed in every case but one

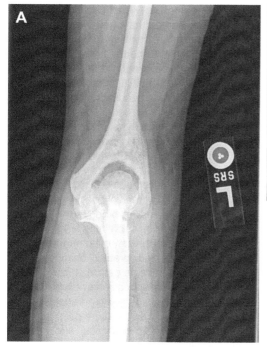

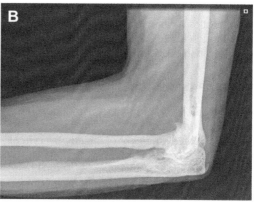

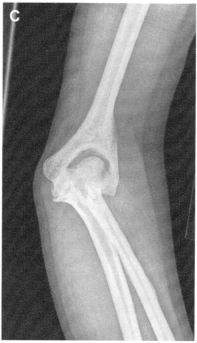

Fig. 1. (A–C) Radiographs of the elbow in this 36-year-old man with long-standing untreated hemophilia B and hemophilic arthropathy demonstrate structural changes and arthritis.

with concomitant contralateral knee involvement, suggesting that use of a crutch or a cane in the hand opposite the symptomatic knee may have been causative.[4] In 1 series, elbow arthropathy seemed to be concordant with the severity of lower extremity arthropathy, suggesting that this may be less related to trauma and more related to individual factors.[22]

Despite fairly profound joint changes, some patients find the function of their elbows acceptable and/or may be unwilling to consider surgery.[3,25] In a series of 26 patients with severe arthropathy of the elbow, most had a functional range of motion, and unimpaired activities of daily living, although 6 had severe restriction of motion but still declined surgical management.[3]

RADIOGRAPHIC FEATURES

The incidence of radiographic joint changes in the elbow ranges from 25% to 87%.[22,28] Radiographic findings include enlargement of the epiphysis in all patients and osteoporosis in 95% of patients, as well as subchondral irregularities.[4,22] Radial head enlargement or splaying is commonly observed (**Fig. 2**).[4,29] In 1 series of patients, complete obliteration of the capitello-condylar groove was observed in 52%, while the remaining 48% had some alteration; radial head enlargement or splaying was present in 66.7% in one series.[4] Soft tissue swelling was present in 81% of patients. Widening of the olecranon fossa was seen in 52%, and irregular subchondral surfaces in 71.4%, and narrowing of the joint in 57%, with joint erosions in 43%. Lipping of the medial joint was seen in 62% of patients.[4] Joint deformity, marginal erosions, and subchondral cyst develop as a later finding.[22] No correlation between duration of disease or bleeding score and clinical and radiographic scoring was found in one series.[4] In contrast, most other series suggest severity of arthropathy increases with age, both clinically and radiographically, and there exists a relationship between the number of hemarthroses and the extent of joint destruction, although in a few cases, arthropathy was found after only a few bleeds.[22,29] In some series, it has been noted that radiographic changes were readily apparent before the onset of pain or stiffness and may be profound before or without appreciable loss of motion.[22,25] Approximately half of patients in one series recalled an initial traumatic episode that resulted in the first hemarthrosis, and then after that bleed, there were additional episodes of hemorrhage. About 39% of patients reported this traumatic episode to occur after the age of 10 years, and 24% stated this was after age 20, and this could occur as late as age 51 years.[22] Some patients presented with joint changes in the absence of recalled or clinically documented evident episodes of hemarthrosis; presumably due to forgotten episodes or those that occurred early in life.[29]

Clinical and radiographic classification of hemophilic arthropathy was described by the World Federation of Haemophilia, which includes assessment of pain, incidence and severity of hemarthroses, clinical examination, and radiographic changes.[26] Pain is graded as 0 (no pain, no deficit); 1 (mild pain, does not interfere with use, occasional need for analgesia); 2 (moderate pain, some interference, occasional analgesia required); or 3 (severe pain, frequent use of analgesics [use of narcotics] and interference with normal use). Hemorrhage occurring for more than 1 year is rated grade 0 (none); grade 1 (1–3 minor bleeds, no major bleeds); grade 2 (1–2 major bleeds, 4–6 minor bleeds); grade 3 (≥3 major bleeds, ≥7 minor bleeds); clinical features of swelling (0 = nil, present = 2), muscle atrophy (nil = 0, present = 1), joint crepitus (nil = 0, present = 1), range of motion (<10% loss = 0; 10%–30% loss = 1, >30% loss = 2; flexion contracture <15° = 0; >15° = 2; instability (nil = 0, present but function not affected = 1; present and interferes with function and requires bracing = 2).

Radiographic changes have been described in grading systems (**Tables 1–3**).[5,26,30]

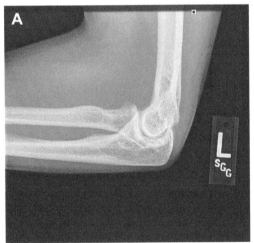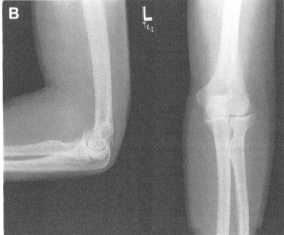

Fig. 2. (*A, B*) Plain films demonstrate splaying of the radial head in this 21-year-old man with hemophila A, which is typical of the hemophilic elbow.

Table 1 Arnold-Hilgartner scale	
Stage	**Findings**
0	Normal joint
I	No skeletal abnormalities; soft tissue swelling present
II	Osteoporosis and overgrowth of epiphysis; no erosions; no narrowing of cartilage space
III	Early subchondral bone cysts; squaring of the patella; intercondylar notch of distal femur or humerus widened; cartilage space remains preserved
IV	Findings of stage III more advanced; cartilage space narrowed
V	Fibrous joint contracture; loss of joint cartilage space; marked enlargement of the epiphysis; and substantial disorganization of the joint

Adapted from Arnold WD, Hilgartner MW. Hemophilic arthropathy. Current concepts of pathogenesis and management. J Bone Joint Surg Am 1977;59:287–305; with permission.

Table 2 Pettersson scale		
Type of Change	**Finding**	**Score**
Osteoporosis	Absent	0
	Present	1
Enlarged epiphysis	Absent	0
	Present	1
Irregular subchondral surface	Absent	0
	Partially involved	1
	Totally involved	2
Narrowing of joint space	Absent	0
	Joint space >1 mm	1
	Joint space <1 mm	2
Subchondral cyst formation	Absent	0
	1 cyst	1
	>1 cyst	2
Erosions of joint margins	Absent	0
	Present	1
Gross incongruence of articulating bone ends	Absent	0
	Slight	1
	Pronounced	2
Joint deformity (angulation and/or displacement between articulating bones)	Absent	0
	Slight	1
	Pronounced	2
Possible joint score:	—	0–13

Adapted from Pettersson H, Ahlberg A, Nilsson IM. A radiologic classification of hemophilic arthropathy. Clin Orthop Relat Res 1980;(149):153–9; with permission.

CLINICAL MANAGEMENT OF HEMOPHILIC ARTHROPLASTY

During the first half of the twentieth century, the life expectancy of those with hemophilia was only 25 to 30 years, and most were severely disabled by age 20 years because of uncontrolled and recurrent hemarthroses. By the 1960s, life expectancy increased to 40 years because of transfusions of whole blood and plasma, but most patients were still severely disabled. The first commercially available plasma-derived clotting factor concentrate was introduced in 1968, and life expectancy for patients with hemophilia increased to 60 years by 1980.[2,31–33] Soon thereafter, the first cases of AIDS were reported in patients with hemophilia and ultimately more than 50% were infected with human immunodeficiency virus (HIV) and more than 75% were infected with viral hepatitis. Since the introduction of virally inactivated factor concentrates in 1985 and the widespread availability and use of recombinant factor products in the 1990s, patients with hemophilia now can lead a normal or near-normal length of life.[2]

At present, attention and objectives of hemophilia management have shifted to prevention of arthropathy and other long-term complications related to bleeding episodes and focus on quality of life issues in the long term.[2] Factor replacement therapy is a mainstay of treatment and is either administered as needed to treat bleeding episodes (on demand) and/or on a scheduled ongoing basis (prophylactically) and/or to prevent bleeding in anticipation of an activity or event likely to provoke bleeding (preventative).[1,2] Factor replacement can come in the form of plasma-derived human or animal products or recombinant products.

Primary prophylaxis refers to initiation of therapy before bleeding episodes with the goal of preventing hemarthroses; secondary prophylaxis is given after hemarthroses have occurred, with the goal of delaying progression of joint arthrosis.[2] The medical and scientific advisory council of the National Hemophilia Foundation, the World Federation of Hemophilia, and the World Health Organization have all recommended prophylactic factor infusion to prevent bleeding episodes and the development of secondary sequelae such as arthropathy as standard of care, as the evidence clearly indicates that prophylaxis, rather than on-demand therapy, is more effective in preventing and delaying arthropathy.[34] In a series of 65

Table 3 Denver magnetic resonance imaging scale	
Score	Findings
0	Normal joint
Effusion/hemarthrosis	
1	Small
2	Moderate
3	Large
Synovial hyperplasia/hemosiderin	
4	Small
5	Moderate
6	Large
Cysts/erosions	
7	1 cyst or partial surface erosion
8	>1 cyst or full surface erosion
Cartilage loss	
9	<50% cartilage loss
10	>50% cartilage loss

Adapted from Nuss R, Kilcoyne RF, Geraghty S, et al. MRI findings in haemophilic joints treated with radiosynoviorthesis with development of an MRI scale of joint damage. Haemophilia 2000;6:162–9; with permission.

children aged 30 monthsor younger with severe hemophilia randomized to on-demand therapy versus prophylaxis, those treated with prophylactic factor replacement therapy had an 83% reduction in risk for joint changes by magnetic resonance imaging (MRI) on follow-up at age 6 years. It has also been suggested that subclinical bleeds or bleeding into the subchondral region may be responsible for joint damage to some extent and this may be lessened by prophylactic therapy but not on-demand therapy.[35] In patients with established arthropathy, secondary prophylactic therapy may still be helpful to decrease the frequency and severity of bleeds.[1] Although factor replacement is costly, there is general consensus that overall primary prophylaxis is cost-effective given that it results in significant improvement in clinical outcomes over the long term, and ultimate factor use is similar when compared with on-demand therapy.[36] Nevertheless, the high cost associated with intensive factor replacement is a barrier to its use for many patients, particularly in underdeveloped countries. Moreover, with the role of primary prophylaxis in adults with hemophilia not yet clearly established, and even with regular factor prophylaxis given during childhood and adolescence, many patients still eventually present with even established or evolving joint changes that are symptomatic.

Physical examination of the hemophilic elbow documents presence of synovitis and malalignment or deformity. Active and passive range of motion are measured with assessment of whether end arc of motion is limited by a hard bony endpoint or a soft endpoint secondary to swelling and pain.[7] Patients are queried about mid arc of motion pain (suggestive of widespread joint abnormalities that may require resurfacing) versus pain only at the end arc of motion (more suggestive of osteophytes that may be removed to improve symptoms).

At least 3 plain-view radiographs of the elbow are taken. Axial imaging, such as MRI, is useful to detect early joint changes and synovitis, and several rating scales have been proposed to describe findings (**Fig. 3**).[7,37] The Denver scale rates MRI findings from 0 to 10, with 0 representing a normal joint, 1 to 3 progressively more effusion and hemarthrosis, 4 to 6 synovial hypertrophy and hemosiderin deposits, 7 to 8 joint erosion and cystic change, and 9 to 10 cartilage loss.[7,37] The European scale of MRI findings is represented by A(e:s:h), with a maximum score of 16(4:4:4). *A* represents a 16-point estimate of bone and cartilage status, including presence of subchondral cysts, erosive changes, and chondral destruction; *e* is a 0 to 4 measurement of effusion or hemarthrosis, *s* is a measure of hypertrophic synovium, and *h* is a 0 to 4 assessment of hemosiderin deposits.[7,37]

Computed tomography scans, particularly with 3-dimensional reconstructions, are helpful for assessment of bony hypertrophic arthritis and in

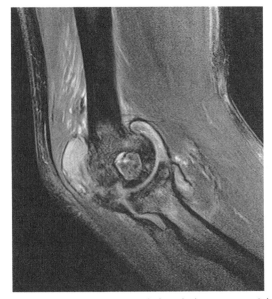

Fig. 3. MRI demonstrates subchondral cysts, synovial hyperplasia and synovitis, and chondral changes in this elbow of a 21-year-old man with hemophilia A.

preparation for surgery, particularly open or arthroscopic debridement (**Fig. 4**).

OPTIONS FOR MANAGEMENT

When approaching patients and taking the history, it is important to consider the number and frequency of bleeds occurring monthly in the affected joint, as well as the pattern and response to factor replacement therapy.[7] Generally, if recurrent bleeds or synovitis is problematic, an initial step is to start intensive factor replacement therapy to stop bleeding and decrease the frequency of recurrent bleeds. Occasionally the joint may respond to a corticosteroid injection to interrupt the cycle by which bleeding-induced inflammation leads to recurrent bleeding. Failure of these measures or symptomatic joint changes, such as

loss of motion or pain, are indications to consider surgery.

An alternative to surgical synovectomy is synoviorthesis, which does not require anesthesia, is not accompanied by surgery, and has lower risk of bleeding complications. Indications include chronic synovitis and recurrent hemarthroses. However, loss of motion can be addressed with synovectomy, whereas motion is unlikely to be substantially improved with synoviorthesis.[7] Synoviorthesis results in ablation of the synovium by injection of chemical or radioactive substances into the joint, which are intended to induce fibrosis of the synovium.[1,38]

Because patients need only to be treated with prophylactic factor dosing for a short time to cover the trauma of this outpatient injection, costs are substantially lower with synoviorthesis compared

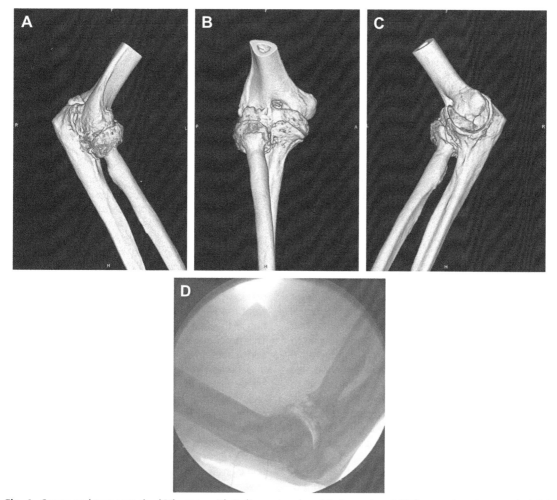

Fig. 4. Computed tomography (CT) scans with 2-dimensional and 3-dimensional (3D) reconstructions are helpful for preoperative planning. This 57-year-old man had right (dominant) hemophilic arthropathy of the elbow and complained most of lack of pronosupination. CT scans with 3D reconstructions (*A–C*) were helpful for preoperative planning before debridement and radial head resection (*D*).

with surgical synovectomy. In 1 series, costs of radioactive synovectomy (RS) were estimated at US $2850 compared with US $61,000 for surgery.[39]

Synoviorthesis may be indicated in patients with a single joint involvement recalcitrant to factor replacement. Ideally, synovial ablation is performed before the development of substantial joint destructive changes. Reported results are 75% to 80% satisfactory in the medium to long term, with reduction in hemoarthroses.[39–43] In some cases, patients may fail to respond adequately to a single injection or recurrent hemarthroses may develop again after an initially successful synoviorthesis; in such cases, treatment may be repeated up to 3 times.[44] Extra-articular extravasation of the materials is a potential risk.[38] Chemical agents for synoviorthesis include osmic acid or rifampin, and radioactive agents include yttrium, gold, or phosphorus.[38,40] Phosphorous 32 has been used in the United States since 1988, although there have been 2 reports of acute lymphoblastic leukemia in young patients less than 12 months after RS.[1,45] Comparative population studies do not seem to demonstrate an increased risk of cancer with use of RS.[1,46] However, the manufacturer of this isotope has recently discontinued production in the United States and it is no longer available.

Although chemical or RS is effective in reducing bleeds, it does nothing for joint incongruity or articular changes or lack of motion. In such cases, surgical management may be a better option. In addition, surgical synovectomy can be considered if synoviorthosis fails.

SURGICAL SYNOVECTOMY AND DEBRIDEMENT

Indications for surgical synovectomy and debridement include failure of 6 months or more of factor replacement prophylaxis to adequately control recurrent hemarthroses or chronic synovitis. Pain and/or motion deficit are also indications to consider this procedure.[7] Severe degenerative changes are a relative contraindication because painful severe joint changes may not respond to debridement alone and might require joint resurfacing such as arthroplasty. Inability to obtain adequate hemostasis, such as presence of an inhibitor antibody to infused clotting factors, is also considered a contraindication.[7]

After synovectomy or debridement, the best predictor of outcomes seems to be the amount of joint changes present on preoperative imaging studies and intraoperative assessment of cartilage changes.[7] Dunn and colleagues[47] noted that bleeding frequency decreased by 85% and motion

remained stable or improved. Journeycake and colleagues[48] evaluated knee, ankle, and elbow arthroscopic synovectomies with stable or improved motion postoperatively and noted fewer hemarthroses at 1 year, which was maintained in 23 of 26 cases at 5 years. However, progression of joint changes does not seem to be halted with synovectomy.[6,47] Synovectomy may be performed by arthroscopic or open means. Both procedures seem to be successful in limiting bleeding episodes and improving pain and motion, and as for other indications, either may be chosen based on experience of surgeon and pathologic condition present.

Post and colleagues[6] reported on open synovectomy for severe hemophilic arthropathy in 17 patients and 5 elbows. The frequency of hemarthroses was greatly decreased postoperatively, especially in the elbow, in which no patients had a bleed postoperatively. The investigators noted that there was a reduced incidence of bleeding; however, the progression of joint changes was not halted. In these patients, synovectomy was performed for frequent or persistent hemorrhage in subacute or early chronic changes that did not respond to factor replacement. For the elbow, a lateral incision at the Kocher interval was performed with radial head resection as indicated. Range of motion was decreased in 4 of these 5 elbows in patients, which may be related to the nature of and compliance with the rehabilitation program postoperatively.[6]

Le Balc'h and colleagues[49] reported on synovectomy of 23 elbows and 18 patients with severe hemophilia. In these patients, preoperatively recurrent and frequent hemoarthroses (at least 2 hemoarthroses per month for 6 months) were recalcitrant to factor replacement therapy and all failed nonoperative treatment, including prophylactic factor replacement (n = 6), intra-articular corticosteroid (n = 4), and osmic acid synoviorthesis (n = 5). Patients underwent medial and lateral incision early in the series, but in the last 8 only a lateral incision was used. This procedure resulted in decreased surgical time, and resection of the radial head was performed in 3 patients. Postoperative complications included hematomas, one on the medial side ultimately requiring ulnar nerve decompression. At mean follow-up of 18 months, 85% of the patients had no bleeds and others had fewer bleeds. Twenty elbows were pain free, and 60% experienced a greater than 10° increase in flexion extension, while pronosupination increased more than 15° in 40% of the elbows. However, flexion decreased more than 15° in 15% of cases, usually older patients. A low rate of complications was seen in this series.

Although hemarthroses are reliably decreased after surgical synovectomy, many of the earlier studies on surgical synovectomy and joint debridement of the elbow demonstrate little improvement and occasional worsening of joint motion; this finding may be related to older rehabilitation protocols involving immobilization to maintain hemostasis. More recent series suggest a beneficial effect on range of motion, particularly with radial head resection.

Silva and colleagues[50] reported on radial head resection and synovectomy for hemophilic arthropathy. A Kocher incision was suggested for anterior synovectomy and resection of the radial head with an oscillating saw just distal to the ulnar facet and proximal to the annular ligament. Posteriorly, the triceps was elevated to perform posterior synovectomy and debridement. Unless concomitant joint debridement of anterior osteophytes and posterior impinging osteophytes is performed, flexion-extension arc is unlikely to improve after radial head resection alone.[50]

Gamble and colleagues[27] described long-term follow-up at average of 10.6 years in 3 patients (4 elbows) in whom synovectomy and radial head excision was performed for elbow pain, recurrent bleeding, or arthrosis at the radiocapitellar joint at an average age of 22 years. Pronation and supination improved and elbow bleeding and pain decreased substantially.

Arthroscopic synovectomy for hemophilia involves a similar procedure to that for other indications. The capsule may be thickened and fibrotic, and a capsulotomy or capsulectomy may be performed. Radial head resection may be performed arthroscopically if indicated.[7] Arthroscopic synovectomy was reported on by Dunn and colleagues[47] in 44 pediatric patients (21 elbows). In this series, patients were indicated for synovectomy either because of failure of medical management or long-term effusion lasting more than 4 months, or late arthritic changes. Patients had less bleeding incidences, and range of motion seemed to be preserved or slightly improved. However, as noted in prior studies of open procedures for synovectomy, radiographic progression of arthrosis was still noted.

JOINT REPLACEMENT ARTHROPLASTY

Butler-Manuel and colleagues[51] investigated silastic interposition arthroplasty for hemophilic arthropathy of the elbow in 13 elbows (12 patients). In follow-up averaging 6.75 years, all 13 elbows had improvement in level of pain and fewer intra-articular bleeding episodes. Moreover, the investigators reported an increase of 20° in the flexion and extension arc and an increase of 62° in prono-supination. Revision for infection was required in

3 elbows(n = 1) or fragmentation of the silastic prosthesis (n = 2).[51] Reduction in cost because of decreased need for factor replacement therapy was found after silastic joint replacement in addition to improved motion, decreased pain, and fewer hemoarthroses.[51,52] However, concerns over durability and silicone synovitis limit use of this implant.

Encouraging results after total elbow arthroplasty for fracture or rheumatoid arthritis have expanded the use of total elbow arthroplasty. Limited data regarding results in the setting of hemophilic arthropathy are available. However, existing data suggest a role for elbow replacement arthroplasty in the hemophilic elbow.

The results of total elbow arthroplasty in a series of 7 elbows in 5 patients with severe hemophilia A at a mean 42 months of follow-up was described by Chapman-Sheath and colleagues.[53] The average age of patients was 48 years. Improved pain, range of motion, and function were noted in all patients; however, complications included one ulnar nerve palsy, an axillary vein thrombosis, and a case of septic loosening requiring debridement and revision.[53]

Kamineni and colleagues[54] also have reported results after total elbow joint replacement arthroplasty. Over a 23-year period, only 5 patients at a large referral center underwent elbow arthroplasty for hemophilic arthropathy of the elbow.[54] The investigators highlighted several issues of concern in this patient population. In addition to the difficulties posed by their underlying bleeding tendency, all 5 patients had HIV infection, and 2 had hepatitis C virus infection. In this series, 3 of 5 patients had a significant complication. In 1 patient who also had an inhibitor antibody, uncontrollable hemorrhage at the surgical site necessitated a return to the operating room on the same day of surgery; although no discrete bleeders were identified, the wound was packed for hemostasis and then closed. After 2 months, the patient presented with wound necrosis and deep infection, which failed to respond to serial debridement but did respond to rotational flap coverage and resection arthroplasty. A second patient developed a deep infection at 4 years postoperatively, and in this case, the implant could be salvaged.[54] One patient complained of persistent pain postoperatively, whereas a second patient experienced recurrent intra-articular bleeds.[54]

Kamineni and colleagues[54] highlighted the difficulties associated with the intraoperative course in these patients. Differences in anatomy should be expected; in 1 case the humeral and ulnar canals were sclerotic and obliterated, and placement of reamers and prostheses required use of high-speed drills for canal preparation, whereas a second patient had a very small canal requiring additional care for placement of the prosthesis.[54] In the 4 patients who retained their implants, functional results according to the MEP score were good (n = 1) or excellent (n = 3) at an average follow-up of 10 years.[54]

OTHER OPTIONS

Other options to consider include interposition arthroplasty, resection arthroplasty, hemiarthroplasty, or fusion. Resection arthroplasty alone results in instability or diminished motion.[55] There were 2 cases of metallic hemiarthroplasty that were described for hemophilic arthropathy but they resulted in ankylosed elbows.[56] Fusion may provide pain relief, with the caveat that function is sacrificed, and it may aggravate adjacent or contralateral joint arthropathy.

PREOPERATIVE AND PERIOPERATIVE CONSIDERATIONS

Preoperatively, each patient should be assessed for the presence of an inhibitor because they present unique challenges in the context of surgery.[7] If inhibitor titers are low, the presence of the inhibitor may be overcome with higher doses of factor. However, for patients with high titer inhibitors, standard factor replacement therapy is not an option, and they must be treated with prothrombin complex concentrates or recombinant factor VIIa.[1,57,58] These "bypassing agents" have less predictable and complete efficacy, they cannot be monitored with standard laboratory assays, and they are more thrombogenic than standard factor replacement therapy. However, patients with hemophilia with inhibitors typically have advanced arthropathy, often in more than 1 joint. Expertise in the surgical management of such patients is limited to those centers with well-established hemophilia programs and requires a highly coordinated multidisciplinary team approach.

In addition to assessing for the presence of an inhibitor, other preoperative studies should include measurement of platelet count, international normalized ratio (INR), and fibrinogen activity.[59] These measurements are particularly important for patients with liver disease related to chronic viral hepatitis, a common finding in older adults with hemophilia.

Perioperative factor replacement can be accomplished with bolus or continuous factor infusions. Although the minimum factor levels needed to provide effective baseline hemostasis are considered to be 20% to 40%, the goal level in the surgical patient is 80% to 100%. Bolus infusion factor to achieve factor levels of approximately 100% is performed preoperatively followed by additional boluses or continuous factor infusion to maintain circulating levels at 80% to 100% and to maintain them at that level for several days postoperatively. Thereafter, factor levels are typically maintained at 50% to 80% for an additional week. Treatment with factor before physiotherapy sessions is important to help avoid provoking delayed postoperative hemorrhage, and prophylactic factor may be continued for 1 to 3 months postoperatively.

AUTHORS' PREFERRED STRATEGY

Patients with hemophilic arthropathy of the elbow are managed with a multidisciplinary approach under the supervision of a hematologist and hemophilia center interested and experienced with these patients and their needs. In the authors' center, patients are seen by the hemophilia center, including by physical and/or occupational therapists, and routine assessment of motion and joint status is made, including range of motion and status of all major joints. Patients who experience recurrent intra-articular bleeds may be candidates for intensive prophylactic therapy. However, failure of prophylactic factor replacement to control bleeds is an indication to consider other management strategies. Corticosteroid injection alone may provide pain relief and some decrease in synovitis; the injection is covered with factor replacement before the procedure. Synoviorthesis may be considered by chemical or surgical means; synovial ablation alone may decrease the frequency and severity of bleeds but is unlikely to alter joints that have limited motion or painful arthritic changes. Moreover, radioisotopes are now of limited availability at the authors' center; the authors have no personal experience with chemical synovectomy. Arthroscopic or open debridement may decrease bleeding frequency and also address impingement, loose bodies, or early arthritic changes. When joint changes are profound, patients are unlikely to benefit from debridement alone to resolve lack of motion or pain; joint replacement arthroplasty may be considered, with acknowledgment of the limitations placed on use of the arm and the high complication rate (**Fig. 5**).

For cases in which surgery is considered, there is acknowledgment that the surgical intervention itself and the perioperative care are complicated. Risk to the patient and surgical staff should not be underestimated. Many of these patients have acquired blood-borne infections, such as HIV and hepatitis B or C, during the course of the disease and its treatment. It is prudent to avoid passing instruments as much as possible, and to

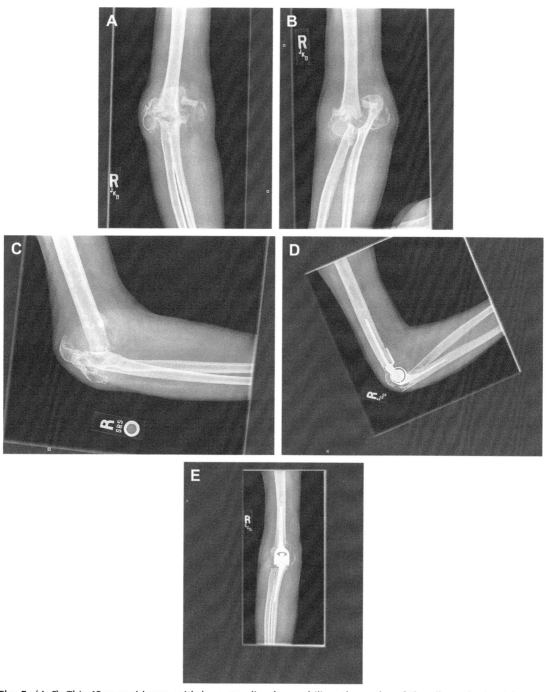

Fig. 5. (*A–E*): This 48-year-old man with long-standing hemophilic arthropathy of the elbows had satisfactory function until he fell, sustaining a fracture of his thinned humeral condyles. His elbow became unstable and painful, and he required a total elbow arthroplasty for relief.

consider the use of face shields, double gloves, or puncture-resistant gloves, and avoid hand-to-hand transmission of instruments, especially sharp instruments.[54] Presence of HIV infection may predispose to a higher rate of wound infections, and HIV-positive status has been associated with a 3-fold higher rate of knee infections postoperatively.[60] As discussed previously, patients with inhibitor antibodies pose an additional set of unique challenges.

Although much progress has been made in the treatment of hemophilia over the last 25 years, hemophilic arthropathy is still a major cause of morbidity, the prevention and management of which is expected to remain a challenge for the foreseeable future, particularly as the hemophilia population ages.

SUMMARY

Hemophilia is a hereditary disease in which circulating levels of coagulation factors are lacking, resulting in a propensity toward bleeding. Intra-articular hemorrhages are a hallmark of hemophilia and may lead a cascade of cytokine elaboration and inflammatory-mediated changes, which ultimately result in cartilage loss and arthropathy. Diarthrodial joints, such as the knee, elbow, and ankle, are most commonly affected. This article highlights issues surrounding hemophilic arthropathy of the elbow and focuses on preventive measures, management strategies of the hemophilic elbow, and treatment options for established arthropathy.

REFERENCES

1. Rodriguez NI, Hoots WK. Advances in hemophilia: experimental aspects and therapy. Pediatr Clin North Am 2008;55:357–76, viii.
2. Rossbach HC. Review of antihemophilic factor injection for the routine prophylaxis of bleeding episodes and risk of joint damage in severe hemophilia A. Vasc Health Risk Manag 2010;6:59–68.
3. Utukuri MM, Goddard NJ. Haemophilic arthropathy of the elbow. Haemophilia 2005;11:565–70.
4. Malhotra R, Gulati MS, Bhan S. Elbow arthropathy in hemophilia. Arch Orthop Trauma Surg 2001;121:152–7.
5. Arnold WD, Hilgartner MW. Hemophilic arthropathy. Current concepts of pathogenesis and management. J Bone Joint Surg Am 1977;59:287–305.
6. Post M, Watts G, Telfer M. Synovectomy in hemophilic arthropathy. A retrospective review of 17 cases. Clin Orthop Relat Res 1986;202:139–46.
7. Verma N, Valentino LA, Chawla A. Arthroscopic synovectomy in haemophilia: indications, technique and results. Haemophilia 2007;13(Suppl 3):38–44.
8. Rodriguez-Merchan EC. Effects of hemophilia on articulations of children and adults. Clin Orthop Relat Res 1996;328:7–13.
9. VanMeegeren M. Update on pathogenesis of the bleeding joint: an interplay between inflammatory and degenerative pathways. Haemophilia 2010;16(Suppl 5):121–3.
10. Fischer K, van der Bom JG, Mauser-Bunschoten EP, et al. The effects of postponing prophylactic treatment on long-term outcome in patients with severe hemophilia. Blood 2002;99:2337–41.
11. Jansen NW, Roosendaal G, Bijlsma J, et al. Exposure of human cartilage tissue to low concentrations of blood for a short period of time leads to prolonged cartilage damage: An in vitro study. Arthritis Rheum 2007;56:199–207.
12. Ovlisen K, Kristensen AT, Jensen AL, et al. IL-1 beta, IL-6, KC and MCP-1 are elevated in synovial fluid from haemophilic mice with experimentally induced haemarthrosis. Haemophilia 2009;15:802–10.
13. Hooiveld M, Roosendaal G, Vianen M, et al. Blood-induced joint damage: longterm effects in vitro and in vivo. J Rheumatol 2003;30:339–44.
14. Hilgartner MW. Current treatment of hemophilic arthropathy. Curr Opin Pediatr 2002;14:46–9.
15. Rodriguez-Merchan EC. Pathogenesis, early diagnosis, and prophylaxis for chronic hemophilic synovitis. Clin Orthop Relat Res 1997;343:6–11.
16. Roosendaal G, TeKoppele JM, Vianen ME, et al. Blood-induced joint damage: a canine in vivo study. Arthritis Rheum 1999;42:1033–9.
17. Roosendaal G, Vianen ME, Marx JJ, et al. Blood-induced joint damage: a human in vitro study. Arthritis Rheum 1999;42:1025–32.
18. Roosendaal G, Vianen ME, van den Berg HM, et al. Cartilage damage as a result of hemarthrosis in a human in vitro model. J Rheumatol 1997;24:1350–4.
19. Hooiveld M, Roosendaal G, Wenting M, et al. Short-term exposure of cartilage to blood results in chondrocyte apoptosis. Am J Pathol 2003;162:943–51.
20. Hooiveld MJ, Roosendaal G, Jacobs KM, et al. Initiation of degenerative joint damage by experimental bleeding combined with loading of the joint: a possible mechanism of hemophilic arthropathy. Arthritis Rheum 2004;50:2024–31.
21. Wallny T, Hess L, Seuser A, et al. Pain status of patients with severe haemophilic arthropathy. Haemophilia 2001;7:453–8.
22. Hogh J, Ludlam CA, Macnicol MF. Hemophilic arthropathy of the upper limb. Clin Orthop Relat Res 1987;218:225–31.
23. Houghton GR, Duthie RB. Orthopedic problems in hemophilia. Clin Orthop 1979;138:197–216.
24. Heim M, Horoszowski H, Martinowitz U, et al. Haemophiliac hands–a three year follow-up study. Hand 1982;14:333–6.
25. Johnson RP, Babbitt DP. Five stages of joint disintegration compared with range of motion in hemophilia. Clin Orthop Relat Res 1985;201:36–42.
26. Pettersson H, Ahlberg A, Nilsson IM. A radiologic classification of hemophilic arthropathy. Clin Orthop Relat Res 1980;149:153–9.
27. Gamble JG, Vallier H, Rossi M, et al. Loss of elbow and wrist motion in hemophilia. Clin Orthop Relat Res 1996;328:94–101.
28. MacDonald PB, Locht RC, Lindsay D, et al. Haemophilic arthropathy of the shoulder. J Bone Joint Surg Br 1990;72:470–1.

29. Wood K, Omer A, Shaw MT. Haemophilic arthropathy. A combined radiological and clinical study. Br J Radiol 1969;42:498–505.

30. Nuss R, Kilcoyne RF, Geraghty S, et al. MRI findings in haemophilic joints treated with radiosynoviorthesis with development of an MRI scale of joint damage. Haemophilia 2000;6:162–9.

31. Chorba TL, Holman RC, Strine TW, et al. Changes in longevity and causes of death among persons with hemophilia A. Am J Hematol 1994;45:112–21.

32. Ikkala E, Helske T, Myllyla G, et al. Changes in the life expectancy of patients with severe haemophilia A in Finland in 1930–79. Br J Haematol 1982;52:7–12.

33. Mejia-Carvajal C, Czapek EE, Valentino LA. Life expectancy in hemophilia outcome. J Thromb Haemost 2006;4:507–9.

34. Berntorp E, Michiels JJ. A healthy hemophilic patient without arthropathy: from concept to clinical reality. Semin Thromb Hemost 2003;29:5–10.

35. Manco-Johnson MJ, Abshire TC, Shapiro AD, et al. Prophylaxis versus episodic treatment to prevent joint disease in boys with severe hemophilia. N Engl J Med 2007;357:535–44.

36. Fischer K, van der Bom JG, Molho P, et al. Prophylactic versus on-demand treatment strategies for severe haemophilia: a comparison of costs and long-term outcome. Haemophilia 2002;8:745–52.

37. Lundin B, Ljung R, Pettersson H. MRI scores of ankle joints in children with haemophilia–comparison with clinical data. Haemophilia 2005;11:116–22.

38. Rodriguez-Merchan EC, Goddard NJ. The technique of synoviorthesis. Haemophilia 2001;7(Suppl 2):11–5.

39. Silva M, Luck JV Jr, Seigel M. 32P chromic phosphate radiosynovectomy for chronic haemophilic synovitis. Haemophilia 2001;7(Suppl 2):40–9.

40. Caviglia HA, Fernandez-Palazzi F, Galatro G, et al. Chemical synoviorthesis with rifampicin in haemophilia. Haemophilia 2001;7(Suppl 2):26–30.

41. Rivard GE, Girard M, Belanger R, et al. Synoviorthesis with colloidal 32P chromic phosphate for the treatment of hemophilic arthropathy. J Bone Joint Surg Am 1994;76:482–8.

42. Rodriguez-Merchan EC, Quintana M, De la Corte-Rodriguez H, et al. Radioactive synoviorthesis for the treatment of haemophilic synovitis. Haemophilia 2007;13(Suppl 3):32–7.

43. Rodriguez-Merchan EC, Wiedel JD. General principles and indications of synoviorthesis (medical synovectomy) in haemophilia. Haemophilia 2001; 7(Suppl 2):6–10.

44. Luck JV Jr, Silva M, Rodriguez-Merchan EC, et al. Hemophilic arthropathy. J Am Acad Orthop Surg 2004;12:234–45.

45. Manco-Johnson MJ, Nuss R, Lear J, et al. 32P Radiosynoviorthesis in children with hemophilia. J Pediatr Hematol Oncol 2002;24:534–9.

46. Infante-Rivard C. Is there an increased risk of cancer associated with radiosynoviorthesis? Haemophilia 2006;12:8–13.

47. Dunn AL, Busch MT, Wyly JB, et al. Arthroscopic synovectomy for hemophilic joint disease in a pediatric population. J Pediatr Orthop 2004;24:414–26.

48. Journeycake JM, Miller KL, Anderson AM, et al. Arthroscopic synovectomy in children and adolescents with hemophilia. J Pediatr Hematol Oncol 2003;25:726–31.

49. Le Balc'h T, Ebelin M, Laurian Y, et al. Synovectomy of the elbow in young hemophilic patients. J Bone Joint Surg Am 1987;69:264–9.

50. Silva M, Luck JV Jr. Radial head excision and synovectomy in patients with hemophilia. Surgical technique. J Bone Joint Surg Am 2008;90(Suppl 2 Pt 2):254–61.

51. Butler-Manuel PA, Smith MA, Savidge GF. Silastic interposition for haemophilic arthropathy of the elbow. J Bone Joint Surg Br 1990;72:472–4.

52. Smith MA, Savidge GF, Fountain EJ. Interposition arthroplasty in the management of advanced haemophilic arthropathy of the elbow. J Bone Joint Surg Br 1983;65:436–40.

53. Chapman-Sheath PJ, Giangrande P, Carr AJ. Arthroplasty of the elbow in haemophilia. J Bone Joint Surg Br 2003;85:1138–40.

54. Kamineni S, Adams RA, O'Driscoll SW, et al. Hemophilic arthropathy of the elbow treated by total elbow replacement. A case series. J Bone Joint Surg Am 2004;86:584–9.

55. Dickson RA, Stein H, Bentley G. Excision arthroplasty of the elbow in rheumatoid disease. J Bone Joint Surg Br 1976;58:227–9.

56. Street DM, Stevens PS. A humeral replacement prosthesis for the elbow: results in ten elbows. J Bone Joint Surg Am 1974;56:1147–58.

57. Hedner U. Treatment of patients with factor VIII and factor IX inhibitors with special focus on the use of recombinant factor VIIa. Thromb Haemost 1999;82:531–9.

58. O'Connell N, Mc Mahon C, Smith J, et al. Recombinant factor VIIa in the management of surgery and acute bleeding episodes in children with haemophilia and high responding inhibitors. Br J Haematol 2002;116:632–5.

59. Ingerslev J, Hvid I. Surgery in hemophilia. The general view: patient selection, timing, and preoperative assessment. Semin Hematol 2006; 43:S23–6.

60. Ragni MV, Crossett LS, Herndon JH. Postoperative infection following orthopaedic surgery in human immunodeficiency virus-infected hemophiliacs with CD4 counts < or = 200/mm3. J Arthroplasty 1995; 10:716–21.

Osteocapsular Debridement for Elbow Arthritis

Leonid I. Katolik, MD

KEYWORDS

- Osteocapsular debridement • Olecranon process
- Elbow arthritis • Osteophyte

Primary osteoarthritis of the elbow, with pain, limitation of motion to within a 30° to 110° arc of flexion and extension, and resistance to nonoperative interventions, is well indicated for treatment by osteocapsular debridement. Initial management of primary elbow arthritis consists of activity modification, antiinflammatory medication, intra-articular injection, and, occasionally, therapy. When these modalities prove unsuccessful, surgical intervention may be warranted if symptoms persist. Given the generally young age and high functional demand of patients with primary osteoarthritis of the elbow, prosthetic replacement is generally not recommended. Joint debridement and release has traditionally been the primary surgical option for the treatment of these patients because the central ulnohumeral joint space is typically maintained. Total joint replacement is reserved for individuals with more advanced arthrosis with lower functional demands who are older than 60 to 65 years.

Individuals with primary arthritis of the elbow typically have bony overgrowth and osteophytes at the coronoid and olecranon processes, respectively. Fluffy densities may be observed filling the olecranon and coronoid fossae, and loose bodies can be seen. Narrowing at the radiocapitellar joint is a common finding. This joint may be the "wear generator" in many patients despite a lack of pain specifically during forearm rotation. The central aspect of the ulnohumeral joint is characteristically spared in this patient population. Pain throughout the arc of elbow motion usually signifies synovitis or articular cartilage degeneration in the central ulnohumeral articulation. This condition is rare and only seen in late disease.

Up to 20% of patients with primary osteoarthritis of the elbow have some degree of ulnar neuropathy. The close association of the nerve to the posteromedial joint capsule leaves it susceptible to impingement from osteophytes or medial joint synovitis expanding the capsule. Early cubital tunnel syndrome in these patients may often manifest as pain at the medial elbow. It is thus important to examine these individuals for signs of ulnar nerve irritability and traction.

PATIENT EVALUATION

Patients with advanced primary osteoarthritis of the elbow present with pain. The pain is typically worse at end flexion and end extension because of the impingement of coronoid or olecranon osteophytes against an overgrown coronoid fossa or olecranon fossa, respectively. Motion is typically limited in all these patients with loss of terminal extension and flexion compared with a normal age- and gender-matched cohort. Most patients have bilateral disease, and as such, the contralateral limb often does not serve as a good "normal" comparison. In the author's practice, loss of motion beyond a flexion extension arc of 30° to 110° qualifies patients with these symptoms for consideration for open capsular debridement. Pain and mechanical symptoms in the setting of maintained range of motion warrant consideration of arthroscopic release.

Many of these patients have ulnar nerve irritation, which must be documented and often addressed surgically. In the author's practice, patients with less than 90° flexion routinely

The Philadelphia Hand Center, P.C., The Merion Building, Suite 200, 700 South Henderson Road, King of Prussia, PA 19406, USA
E-mail address: likatolik@HANDCENTERS.com

Hand Clin 27 (2011) 165–170
doi:10.1016/j.hcl.2011.03.001

undergo ulnar nerve decompression with osteo-capsular debridement.

Radiographically, the primary pathologic condition of osteoarthritis of the elbow includes the presence of osteophytes of the coronoid and olecranon processes, as well as osteophytic overgrowth of the coronoid and olecranon fossae. Advanced imaging is rarely used in preoperative planning.

TECHNIQUE
Lateral Approach

The lateral approach remains the author's preferred method for capsular debridement. Advantages to the lateral exposure include an internervous subcutaneous plane, simplicity, possibly less muscular morbidity with respect to the extensor and flexor-pronator muscular origin release, and access to all 3 joint articulations, namely, the ulnohumeral, radiocapitellar, and proximal radioulnar joints. The main disadvantage of the lateral exposure is the need to address the ulnar nerve, when indicated, through a separate incision.

From a purely mechanical standpoint, to improve elbow flexion, any soft tissue structure must be released posteriorly, which might be tethering the joint. The structures include the posterior joint capsule as well as the triceps muscle and tendon, which can become adherent to the humerus. In addition, any bony or soft tissue impingement must be removed anteriorly, including osteophytes off of the coronoid process, and any bony or soft tissue overgrowth in both the coronoid and radial fossae. There must be a concavity above the humeral trochlea to accept both the coronoid centrally and the radial head laterally for full flexion to occur. Similarly, to improve elbow extension, posterior impingement must be removed between the olecranon tip and the olecranon fossa. Anteriorly, any tethering soft tissue, namely, the anterior joint capsule, and any adhesions between the brachialis and the humerus must be released.

Under regional anesthesia with a long-acting axillary block, an extended Kocher incision is made beginning along the lateral supracondylar ridge of the humerus and passing distally in the interval between the anconeus and extensor carpi ulnaris (ECU). The anconeus is retracted posteriorly, with dissection performed proximally beneath the lateral epicondyle and along the supracondylar ridge of the humerus, thereby retracting both the anconeus and triceps posteriorly. A triceps tenolysis is performed with an elevator, releasing any adhesions between the muscle and the posterior humerus. The ulnohumeral joint is identified posteriorly and the olecranon fossa cleared of any fibrous tissue or scar, which would restrict terminal extension. The tip of the olecranon is removed if there is evidence of overgrowth or impingement. The posterior aspect of the radiocapitellar joint is inspected after excision of the elbow capsule just proximal to the conjoined lateral collateral and annular ligament complex through the soft spot on the lateral side of the elbow. The proximal edge of this complex lies along the proximal border of the radial head. Once the posterior release is completed, dissection is performed anteriorly, releasing the brachioradialis and extensor carpi radialis longus (ECRL) from the lateral supracondylar ridge of the humerus. The brachialis is then mobilized off the humerus and anterior capsule with an elevator, releasing any adhesions between the muscle and the anterior humerus. This dissection is continued distally between the ECRL and extensor carpi radialis brevis (ECRB), allowing exposure of the anterior capsule, with preservation of the lateral collateral ligament as well as the origins of the ECRB, the extensor digitorum communis and extensor digiti minimi, and the ECU from the lateral epicondyle. Dissection is then performed beneath the elbow capsule between the joint and the brachialis. The capsule is then excised as far as the medial side of the joint. The radial and coronoid fossae are cleared of fibrous tissue, and the tip of the coronoid is removed if overgrowth or impingement is noted in flexion. Loose bodies are removed. With radiocapitellar degeneration, the joint may be debrided or the radial head resected through the anterior capsulectomy using an oscillating saw or osteotome, without dissecting the lateral collateral ligament complex. After release of the anterior capsule, gentle extension of the elbow with applied pressure usually brings the joint out to nearly full extension. In cases of long-standing contracture, the brachialis muscle can be tight inhibiting full terminal elbow extension. This myostatic contracture may be stretched for several minutes during the procedure and typically requires subsequent dedicated physiotherapy (**Fig. 1**).

Medial Approach

The medial approach facilitates access to the posteromedial olecranon osteophytes and ulnar nerve. The principles are, however, identical to those outlined for the lateral approach. The main disadvantage of the medial approach is the inability to access the radial head and capitellum.

A medial skin incision is made, extending from the distal border of pronator teres, curving along the line of the ulnar nerve, and continuing

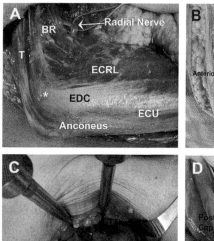

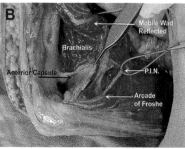

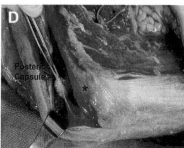

Fig. 1. Anatomy of the lateral approach. (*A*) Cadaveric specimen with lateral anatomy marked. (*B*) ECRL is taken down off of the humerus proximally and elevated off of the anterior capsule distally. The radial nerve in this case is dissected out for reference. (*C*) Anterior capsule is excised, and easy access to the anterior joint from lateral to medial is accomplished. (*D*) With the triceps elevated off of the humerus and the anconeus partially elevated off of the distal humerus, the posterior capsule may be excised, and the posterior joint is cleared of bony overgrowth. BR, brachioradialis; EDC, extensor digitorum communis; PIN, posterior interosseous nerve; T, triceps; *, lateral epicondyle.

proximally to the posterior aspect of the arm. Traversing branches of the medial antebrachial cutaneous nerve are preserved within the fat superficial to the fascia overlying the flexor carpi ulnaris (FCU). The ulnar nerve is located just proximally and released distally beyond the 2 heads of the FCU, which are split apart to uncover the nerve. The motor branches to the FCU and the flexor digitorum profundus branch should be preserved.

Once the ulnar nerve is fully mobilized to permit anterior transposition, the medial joint line is exposed up to the anterior oblique bundle (AOB), and the posterior oblique bundle of the medial collateral ligament (MCL) is excised. The posterior compartment of the elbow is easily accessible posteriorly through the interval between the triceps and the posterior aspect of the humerus. A Cobb elevator is used to elevate the triceps from the posterior distal surface of the humerus, followed by the excision of the posterior capsule. The elbow is extended, and the posterior aspects of the humerus and olecranon fossa are exposed. Olecranon osteophytes or overgrowth of the olecranon fossa is excised.

In the anterior compartment of the forearm, after retracting the anterior skin flap, the superficial flexor muscles of the forearm are visible as they pass directly from their common origin on the medial epicondyle of the humerus. The origin of pronator–common flexor group of muscles may be reflected from the medial epicondyle and retracted distally. Alternatively, an incision may be made through the common flexor tendon. This incision generally passes in the interval between flexor carpi radialis and palmaris longus. A deep narrow retractor is inserted to retract the common flexor muscles medially, laterally, and proximally, allowing visualization of the anterior medial capsule. The AOB of MCL attaches onto the anteroinferior aspect of the medial epicondyle. The posterior oblique bundle attaches onto the posteroinferior aspect of the medial epicondyle and forms the floor of the cubital tunnel. With the protection of the AOB by the medial half of the common flexors, the anterior capsule is sharply excised under direct visualization. Once the anterior part of elbow is exposed, any osteophyte from the coronoid process (flexing the elbow) and coronoid fossa (extending the elbow) is removed with a rongeur or chisel, with particular attention to debridement of the anteromedial coronoid without disturbing the anterior portion of the MCL. The radial fossa can be visualized from this point and freed of any osteophyte as needed.

Before wound closure, the ulnar nerve is transposed anteriorly subcutaneously, followed by closure of the wounds in layers over suction drains. A posterior splint is applied with the arm in 70° of flexion.

Posterior Approach

The posterior approach popularized by Outerbridge is uniquely indicated for the small group of patients with impingement and pain at end range of motion, but with relatively good preservation of the overall flexion extension arc beyond 30° to 110°.

A posterior incision is made over the triceps tendon. The triceps is split in the midline to expose the tips of the olecranon and posterior capsule. The capsule is excised to expose the olecranon fossa, which may be opened with a high-speed burr or triple reamer. The coronoid tip comes into view with elbow flexion and may be excised with a rongeur.

The procedure allows for a limited amount of capsular excision and does not allow the surgeon to address ulnar nerve pathology or radiocapitellar disease (**Fig. 2**).

PITFALLS

The most common complication of elbow release surgery involves the ulnar nerve. This complication may, in part, be related to improved elbow flexion after surgery as ulnar nerve tension increases with inflexion. This may precipitate symptoms in a nerve that is already subclinically compromised, if the ulnar nerve is not addressed at time of surgery.

Patients with preoperative signs and symptoms of ulnar nerve irritability should undergo neurolysis and transposition of the ulnar nerve. Although not strict guidelines exist, patients with preoperative flexion less than 90°, generally undergo concurrent ulnar nerve release even in the absence of preoperative symptoms.

The median nerve and brachial artery are at risk with anterior dissection. These structures are generally well protected by the brachialis muscle. The margin of safety is increased if dissection proceeds in the interval between the elbow capsule and the brachialis. Some surgeons find it easiest to elevate the brachialis and ECRL off the humeral ridge and anterior joint capsule with blunt scissors. This author prefers to elevate the ECRL and brachialis off the capsule with a large Cobb elevator. Blunt dissection begins proximally and laterally and extends distally and medially.

Transient median neuritis was found to occur in the author's practice following release. This condition is likely caused by the stretch of the median nerve with extension of the severely contracted elbow.

The posterior interosseous nerve may be encountered as extracapsular dissection proceeds

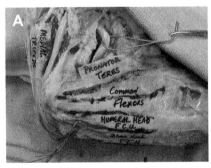
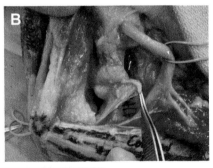
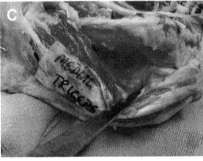

Fig. 2. Anatomy of the posterior approach. (*A*) Cadaveric specimen with the medial anatomy marked. Loops have been placed around the ulnar nerve posteriorly and the median nerve anteriorly. (*B*) The pronator has been reflected off the medial epicondyle. The anterior capsule may be excised. The brachialis muscle is deep in the wound and prevents facile access to the radial fossa and provides no access to the radial head. The median nerve has been dissected for reference. (*C*) The ulnar nerve has been transposed, the medial triceps reflected off of the humerus, and the capsule excised. Wide exposure to the posterior joint is afforded with this approach. (*Courtesy of* Doug Hanel, MD, and Seth Dodds, MD; with permission.)

distal to the radiocapitellar joint. Care must be taken with more distal dissection, and a firm understanding of neural anatomy is mandatory before attempting capsular release. Except in cases of significant anterolateral heterotropic ossification, the radial nerve is not routinely dissected and isolated from proximal to distal.

Finally, the importance of a committed and often prolonged postoperative rehabilitation to prevent stiffness cannot be emphasized enough. A program of active and passive range of motion, weighted elbow stretches with wrist weights, formal therapy, and patient-adjusted elbow bracing is common for 3 to 6 months after surgery. Postoperative gains may easily be lost in patients who are not fully committed to their rehabilitation or who do not have access to regular supervised therapy. At the author's institution, it is recommended that patients meet preoperatively both with the in-house therapists and with their local therapists.

RESULTS

A review of the literature from the last 15 years on open debridement for even advanced primary osteoarthritis of the elbow shows consistent and predictable results from institution to institution. Furthermore, these results are comparable, regardless of the approach (lateral, medial, or posterior) and seem to be durable over a follow-up period of up to 10 years.[1,2]

Oka and colleagues[3] reported a mixed series of lateral, medial, and combined debridements at a mean follow-up period of 6 years. Recurrence of spur formation was identified radiographically in almost all patients but was noted to be minimal. Pain relief was consistent and durable over the follow-up period, whereas gains in motion were only 6° in extension and 18° in flexion. No difference was noted between surgical approaches.

Wada[1] found that the long-term results of debridement via a medial approach were durable at up to 12 years, but with progressive loss of extension. Pain relief and flexion were well maintained.

Kashiwagi[4] reported the results on 111 elbows. There was an improvement of 88% in spontaneous pain and 67% in pain on movement; 76% gained flexion and 55% extension. The mean follow-up period was 5 years.

Modifications of ulnohumeral arthroplasty have been advocated. There has been particular interest in the development of arthroscopic techniques for debridement. Savoie and colleagues[5] reviewed 24 patients who had undergone the procedure arthroscopically, and although encouraging results were obtained, 18 patients had simultaneous excision of the radial head. This was not a feature of the original technique and thus makes comparison with results after the open procedure difficult.

Cohen and colleagues[6] compared arthroscopic ulnohumeral arthroplasty with the open technique. At a mean follow-up period of 35 months, the investigators concluded that the arthroscopic procedure was more effective for pain relief but less effective for improving range of movement.

Both Kashiwagi[4] and Morrey[2] noted that with time, there was recurrent growth of bone at the fenestration of the olecranon fossa. Regrowth of bone and progressive closure of the fenestration of the olecranon fossa may be postulated to be associated with deteriorating function. However, this has not been determined to be the case in these series. No correlation has been found between the functional assessment and the disappearance of the fenestration. This finding is linked to the fact that before operation, the membrane of the olecranon fossa is grossly thickened. Postoperatively, as the fenestration begins to close, regrowth of bone occurs from the circumference of the opening. Although the fenestration may close completely with time, the regrown membrane does not thicken to the same extent as that present preoperatively. This finding suggests that radiologic evidence of recurrent growth of bone and closure of the fenestration of the olecranon fossa are poor indicators for assessing the progress of osteoarthritis of the elbow after ulnohumeral arthroplasty.

SUMMARY

Open capsular debridement is an excellent option for the treatment of elbow arthritis. It is particularly indicated in a patient population physiologically younger than 60 years. It preserves the native joint and thus does not inherently require permanent activity modification as does replacement arthroplasty.

REFERENCES

1. Wada T, Isogai S, Ishii S, et al. Debridement arthroplasty for primary osteoarthritis of the elbow. J Bone Joint Surg Am 2004;86(2):233–41.
2. Morrey BF. Primary degenerative arthritis of the elbow: treatment by ulnohumeral arthroplasty. J Bone Joint Surg Br 1992;74:409–13.
3. Oka Y, Ohta K, Saitoh I. Debridement arthroplasty for osteoarthritis of the elbow. Clin Orthop Relat Res 1998;(351):127–34.

4. Kashiwagi D. Outerbridge-Kashiwagi arthroplasty for osteoarthritis of the elbow in the elbow joint. In: Proceedings of the International Congress, Kobe, Japan. Amsterdam: Excerpta Medica; 1986.

5. Savoie FH 3rd, Nunley PD, Field LD. Arthroscopic management of the arthritic elbow: indications, technique, and results. J Shoulder Elbow Surg 1999;8:214–9.

6. Cohen AP, Redden JF, Stanley D. Treatment of osteoarthritis of the elbow: a comparison of open versus arthroscopic debridement. Arthroscopy 2000;16: 701–6.

Arthroscopy for Arthritis of the Elbow

Felix H. Savoie III, MD[a],*, Michael J. O'Brien, MD[a],
Larry D. Field, MD[b]

KEYWORDS

- Elbow arthroscopy • Elbow arthritis
- Ulnohumeral arthroplasty
- Arthroscopic Outerbridge-Kashiwagi • Fenestration

Degenerative arthritis of the elbow seems to be growing more common and may be a cause of substantial disability.[1–4] Although initially treated nonoperatively, it usually progresses and has been historically managed by open measures. Since the initial report of arthroscopic management of the degenerative elbow by Savoie and colleagues,[5] arthroscopy has become a more common treatment modality, with results comparable to or better than similar open procedures. This report summarizes the current application of arthroscopy for the arthritic elbow.[6–10]

HISTORY AND PHYSICAL EXAMINATION

The cause of primary osteoarthritis of the elbow is usually genetic, but it may occur in manual laborers, athletes, or others whose activities produce excessive stress on the joint.[1–4,11] In addition, injuries of many different kinds, including fractures and dislocation, may produce posttraumatic arthritis.[12]

Symptoms of arthritis include loss of motion, mechanical catching and locking, and pain.[4,11] Pain is usually present at the terminal arc of motion but may occur during any part of movement. Inspection may show deformity and muscle atrophy. Physical examination reveals crepitation, abnormal movement patterns, and a decreased arc of motion. Tenderness may be present over the arthritic deformities and the radiocapitellar articulation and on the epicondyles. Swelling is usually present and may be observed in the lateral gutter. The normal plica on the posterior lateral elbow is usually enlarged and tender.

There may also be spurs present on the medial side, and in some cases, the medial spurs may put pressure on the ulnar nerve. In posttraumatic cases, the nerve may also be tethered by adhesions. In each of these cases, there may be a Tinel sign near the cubital tunnel. The ulnar nerve should always be evaluated in the arthritic elbow for these problems to decrease the incidence of postoperative complications related to the nerve during restoration of motion. Electrical studies may also be useful to document irritation of the ulnar nerve if the clinical examination suggests entrapment or tethering.

DIAGNOSTIC IMAGING

Plain film radiographs should be obtained and they typically demonstrate hypertrophic bony spurs and loose bodies (**Figs. 1** and **2**). The bone is generally sclerotic than osteopenic (as observed in rheumatoid arthritis). Computed tomography (CT) scans may be useful, particularly with 3-dimensional (3D) reconstructions, to map out areas of interest that require recontouring, if this is not readily apparent on the plain radiographs. Using the 3D CT as a preoperative planning tool allows the surgeon to gain an increased

No funding was received relevant to this article by any of the authors.
[a] Department of Orthopaedic Surgery, Tulane University School of Medicine, 1430 Tulane Avenue SL-32, New Orleans, LA 70112-2699, USA
[b] Upper Extremity Service, Mississippi Sports Medicine and Orthopaedic Center, 1325 East Fortification Street, Jackson, MS 39202, USA
* Corresponding author.
E-mail address: busavoie@aol.com

Hand Clin 27 (2011) 171–178
doi:10.1016/j.hcl.2011.01.005

hand.theclinics.com

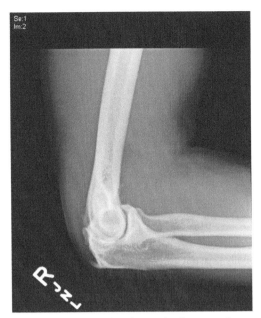

Fig. 1. A typical lateral radiograph of a severely osteoarthritic elbow shows spurs on the coronoid and olecranon processes.

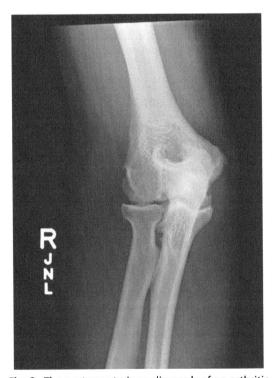

Fig. 2. The posteroanterior radiograph of an arthritic elbow shows sclerotic bone at the radiocapitellar joint and may reveal loose bodies in the coronoid and olecranon fossae.

appreciation for the osteophytic areas that require attention to improve the range of motion and achieve a satisfactory result.

INDICATIONS FOR SURGERY

Nonoperative treatment options, such as nonsteroidal antiinflammatory medications, corticosteroid injections, and activity modifications, should be exhausted before considering surgery.[5] Pain, functional impairment, and a failure of nonoperative treatment are the main indications for surgery. In the arthritic elbow, this indication is usually represented by pain at the end arc of motion, mechanical symptoms, or joint contracture that limits activity. As with all arthritic problems, the main indication for surgery is the decision of the patient, not the physician. Potential problems with surgery involve the ulnar nerve. A subluxating ulnar nerve or a prior subcutaneous ulnar nerve transposition are not necessarily contraindications to arthroscopy of the elbow; however, an intermuscular or submuscular transposition is often considered a relative contraindication unless the precise course of the nerve can be ascertained by visual inspection, palpation, or ultrasonography.

Although the authors think that arthroscopic measures are the best treatment of the arthritic elbow, acceptable alternatives include open procedures, such as resection arthroplasty of the ulnohumeral joint, or open debridement, such as the Morrey ulnohumeral arthroplasty or the Outerbridge-Kashiwagi procedure.[3,4,11–21] In addition, total elbow arthroplasty reliably relieves pain and motion but should be reserved for sedentary individuals with pan-articular changes whose primary complaint is pain, not functional limitation. Arthrodesis of the elbow is reserved for cases in which there is no other option and is often difficult to achieve.[8] At present, given all options, arthroscopic debridement with spur removal and fossa fenestration with or without radial head excision is the preferred treatment because of the ability to address all underlying pathologic processes and provide outcomes similar to, if not better than, open procedures.[5,6,10,22–27]

ARTHROSCOPIC TECHNIQUE

The arthroscopic technique and set up has previously been described and is not repeated here except in general terms.[1,19,20] General or regional anesthesia is induced, and the patient is placed in the prone (authors' preferred method) or lateral decubitus position. All bony prominences are protected. It is useful to use both an eye shield and a protective headrest in the prone position. A

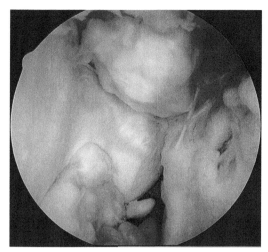

Fig. 3. Arthroscopic view of the coronoid fossa reveals a large loose body.

regular bed sheet, folded into a square and taped securely, can be positioned on the arm board, obviating a special arm holder. This position and bolster allows unrestricted access to the elbow, and the shoulder can be internally or externally rotated to allow access to the medial or lateral elbow. A nonsterile tourniquet is usually applied or a sterile one is used after the arm is prepped and draped in the usual fashion.

Standard equipment for elbow arthroscopy is used. This equipment include the 4-mm 30° arthroscope, interchangeable arthroscopic canulas, retractors, and graspers. Retractors, such as a Freer elevator or a blunt switching stick, are useful to improve the visual field. A standard 3.5 arthroscopic shaver and 4.5 hooded burr are helpful for arthroscopy of the arthritic elbow.

Before insufflation, the path of the ulnar nerve is carefully marked. It is very important that this procedure be done after the patient is positioned because, in the degenerative elbow, the intermuscular septum may be lax and displaced downward by gravity, or the nerve may be subluxated out of the groove in the prone or lateral decubitus position. Marking only the nerve also serves to keep the surgeon oriented to the medial and lateral sides of the elbow.

The joint is distended with 20 to 30 mL saline introduced via an 18-gauge needle through either the posterior central portal or the "soft spot" portal, which is the center of a triangle formed by the olecranon process, the lateral epicondyle, and the radial head. Fluid distention makes portal establishment easier and safer.

Portal sites are tested with a spinal needle, and the opening is made by incising only the skin with the blade. A small (4.0) canula with a blunt trocar is used to enter the joint via a proximal anteromedial portal. If there is difficulty in accessing the joint, then blunt dissection with a hemostat may allow easier access to the capsule and joint. Capsular entry and joint location are confirmed by sudden egress of fluid. The arthroscope is placed into the sleeve, and the joint is evaluated.

ANTERIOR PORTALS

The proximal anterolateral and anteromedial portals are usually used first and are considered safer than the distal anterolateral and anteromedial portals. The proximal anteromedial portal is established first, with care taken to avoid and protect the ulnar nerve. A second anterior portal, the proximal anterolateral portal is then established with an

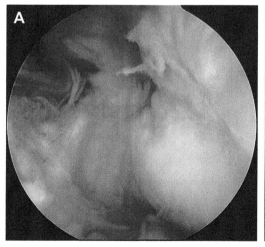

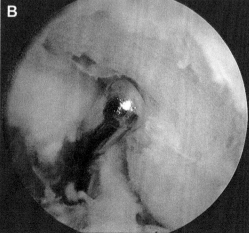

Fig. 4. Arthroscopic view from the proximal anteromedial portal demonstrates the buildup of bone in the radial fossa (*A*) and the view after its excision (*B*).

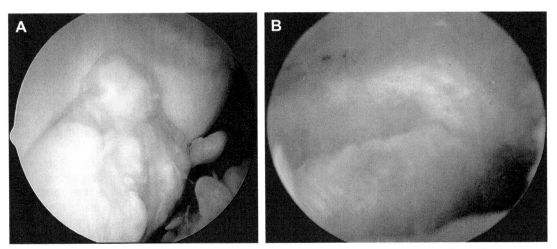

Fig. 5. Commonly seen in the arthritic elbow are large coronoid spurs (*A*). This spur is excised, usually via a shaver in the medial portal (*B*).

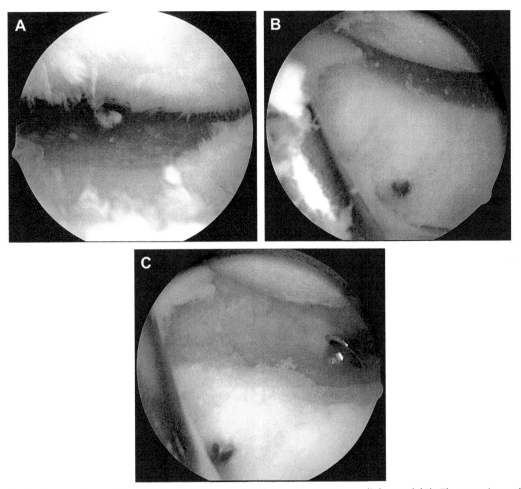

Fig. 6. A degenerative radio capitellar joint is visualized via an anterior medial portal (*A*). The anterior radial head is excised (*B*) first, then the soft spot portal is used to co-plane the resection to a smooth surface (*C*).

outside-in technique. This portal is established just anterior and superior to the most superior aspect of the articular surface of the capitellum to allow access to the radial fossa, if necessary.

ANTERIOR PROCEDURES

Initial inspection of the anterior compartment of an arthritic elbow usually reveals one or more loose bodies, often located in the coronoid fossa (**Fig. 3**). If small, these bodies are removed first, but if large, they may be removed later to preserve joint distension. A 3.5 shaver is used to perform a synovectomy, if necessary. Before switching the scope to the lateral portal, the radial fossa is evaluated (**Fig. 4**A). If necessary, the excess bone is resected to restore the normal anatomy of the radial fossa (see **Fig. 4**B). The spurs on the coronoid are easily visualized from both the proximal medial and lateral portals (**Fig. 5**A) but are more easily removed with the arthroscope in the proximal anterior lateral portal and the shaver in the medial portal (see **Fig. 5**B).

Radial head excision may be necessary in patients with radiocapitellar symptoms, complete loss of cartilage at the radiocapitellar articulation, or significant crepitation with valgus stress during motion. Most easily visualized with the arthroscope in the proximal anteromedial portal, inspection reveals a loss of articular cartilage on both the radial head and capitellum (**Fig. 6**A). Excision of the radial head begins with the burr in the anterior lateral portal to resect the anterior aspect, while protecting the radial nerve (see **Fig. 6**B). The excision is completed via a posterior soft spot portal to allow coplaning to a smooth surface (see **Fig. 6**C), while a retractor is kept in the anterior lateral portal to further protect the radial and posterior interosseous nerves. If there is a loss of motion on pronosupination or pain on pronation and supination, then complete radial head excision past the radial neck may be of benefit. At this time, a fenestration hole connecting the olecranon fossa to the coronoid fossa may be drilled (**Fig. 7**).

POSTERIOR PORTAL PLACEMENT

After the anterior work is completed, an inflow canula is left anteriorly and the posterior aspect of the joint is addressed as indicated. The ulnar nerve should have already been marked and its location should be reconfirmed at this point to prevent injury.

The posterocentral portal is the initial viewing portal and is made with the elbow at 90° flexion. The portal site is placed 3 cm above the tip of the olecranon in the center of the olecranon fossa. The initial view shows considerable spur

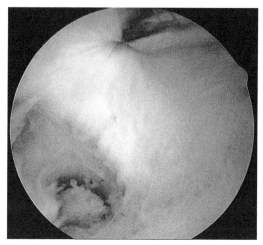

Fig. 7. An anterior view of the drill bit used for connecting the radial and coronoid fossa.

formation in the fossa as well as loose bodies and synovitis (**Fig. 8**). A posterolateral portal is made parallel to this site just outside the triceps tendon. Once the olecranon fossa is cleared and the triceps elevated, the arthroscope is switched to the lateral portal, and the direct posterocentral portal becomes the working portal.

Subsequently, osteophytes are removed from the tip and sides of the olecranon and the rim of the olecranon fossa. The authors have found it useful to drill a fenestration hole in the center of the olecranon fossa and connect it to the coronoid fossa. This drilling allows measuring of the thickness of the bone bridge between the 2 fossae,

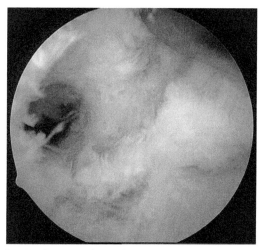

Fig. 8. The view from the posterior portal demonstrating the severe osteophyte formation in the olecranon fossa commonly seen in the degenerative elbow.

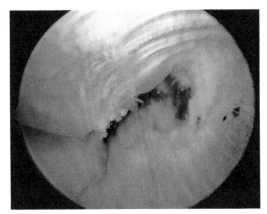

Fig. 9. The posterolateral portal view of a large plica observed on the lateral gutter, a common finding in the degenerative elbow.

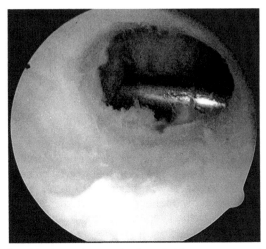

Fig. 11. An arthroscopic Outerbridge procedure is performed by enlargement of the olecranon to coronoid fossa fenestration, with removal of all associated spurs.

which is usually thickened in the arthritic elbow. The fenestration hole also allows improved flow from the anterior canula into the posterior aspect of the elbow.

Once the posterior debridement is complete, the lateral gutter should be evaluated for loose bodies and an enlarged plica (**Fig. 9**). The medial gutters should similarly be debrided of plica and spurs, while protecting the ulnar nerve (**Fig. 10**). The fenestration hole in the fossa is then enlarged to 1 to 2 cm diameter and all fossa spurs excised to complete an arthroscopic Outerbridge procedure (**Fig. 11**). The olecranon tip is then broadly excised until full extension can be achieved (**Fig. 12**). In patients with a profound loss of

motion, the ulnar nerve may also be carefully released by either open or arthroscopic measures (**Fig. 13**).

POSTOPERATIVE REHABILITATION

After completion of the procedure, motion is assessed in the operating room to ensure adequate restoration. Radiographs or fluoroscopy may be used to confirm spur resection and the absence of any additional loose bodies. A drain is placed through the anterior canula and removed before the patient goes home. The portals are closed in the standard fashion with 3-0 sutures, and a sterile compressive dressing is applied.

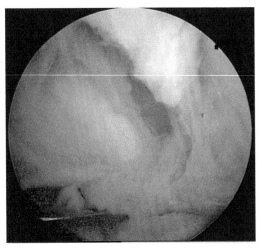

Fig. 10. A less commonly seen pathologic medial plica in a degenerative elbow, showing the changes on the bone of the medial olecranon, the medial humerus, the large medial synovial plica, and the ulnar nerve.

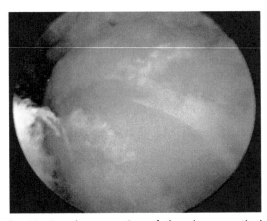

Fig. 12. Complete resection of the olecranon tip is done after the fossa debridement is completed, with medial to lateral resection continued until full extension is achieved.

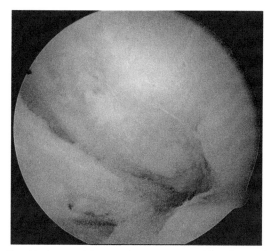

Fig. 13. In special cases for surgeons with advanced skills, the ulnar nerve may be released using arthroscopic techniques as observed, in which the nerve can be seen after being freed from the overlying medial epicondyle.

Range of motion exercise is started on the first postoperative day. No limitations are placed on use of the arm.

Heterotopic ossification (HO) prophylaxis is used in patients with previous problems with HO or in revision cases, consisting of a single dose of 700 cGy radiation therapy within the 48 hours time frame of the procedure. The authors have found that this complication is rarely indicated in patients undergoing primary arthroscopic debridement of the arthritic elbow.

Continuous passive motion may be initiated using a continuous passive motion device, with or without a nerve block, and has been found to be beneficial in patients. The best therapy is to simply begin the active use of the arm through a full arc of motion.

SUMMARY

Arthroscopic spur excision and ulnohumeral arthroplasty for arthritis is an excellent procedure for the treatment of elbow osteoarthritis. Increasing data are becoming available, and it seems that the results and complications are similar if not an improvement, to those of open procedures.

REFERENCES

1. Stanley D. Prevalence and etiology of symptomatic elbow osteoarthritis. J Shoulder Elbow Surg 1994; 3:386–9.

2. Redden JF, Stanley D. Arthroscopic fenestration of the olecranon fossa in the treatment of osteoarthritis of the elbow. Arthroscopy 1993;9(1):14–6.

3. Tsuge K, Mizuseki T. Debridement arthroplasty for advanced primary osteoarthritis of the elbow. Results of a new technique used for 29 elbows. J Bone Joint Surg Br 1994;76(4):641–6.

4. Antuna SA, Morrey BF, Adams RA, et al. Ulnohumeral arthroplasty for primary degenerative arthritis of the elbow: long-term outcome and complications. J Bone Joint Surg Am 2002;84(12):2168–73.

5. Savoie FH 3rd, Nunley PD, Field LD. Arthroscopic management of the arthritic elbow: indications, technique, and results. J Shoulder Elbow Surg 1999; 8(3):214–9.

6. Adams JE, Wolff LH 3rd, Merten SM, et al. Osteoarthritis of the elbow: results of arthroscopic osteophyte resection and capsulectomy. J Shoulder Elbow Surg 2008;17(1):126–31.

7. Ball CM, Meunier M, Galatz LM, et al. Arthroscopic treatment of post-traumatic elbow contracture. J Shoulder Elbow Surg 2002;11(6):624–9.

8. Clasper JC, Carr AJ. Arthroscopy of the elbow for loose bodies. Ann R Coll Surg Engl 2001;83(1):34–6.

9. Cohen AP, Redden JF, Stanley D. Treatment of osteoarthritis of the elbow: a comparison of open and arthroscopic debridement. Arthroscopy 2000; 16(7):701–6.

10. O'Driscoll SW. Arthroscopic treatment for osteoarthritis of the elbow. Orthop Clin North Am 1995; 26(4):691–706.

11. Morrey BF. Primary degenerative arthritis of the elbow. Treatment by ulnohumeral arthroplasty. J Bone Joint Surg Br 1992;74(3):409–13.

12. Suvarna SK, Stanley D. The histologic changes of the olecranon fossa membrane in primary osteoarthritis of the elbow. J Shoulder Elbow Surg 2004; 13(5):555–7.

13. Oka Y, Ohta K, Saitoh I. Debridement arthroplasty for osteoarthritis of the elbow. Clin Orthop Relat Res 1998;351:127–34.

14. Tan V, Daluiski A, Simic P, et al. Outcome of open release for post-traumatic elbow stiffness. J Trauma 2006;61(3):673–8.

15. Mansat P, Morrey BF. The column procedure: a limited lateral approach for extrinsic contracture of the elbow. J Bone Joint Surg Am 1998;80(11):1603–15.

16. Sarris I, Riano FA, Goebel F, et al. Ulnohumeral arthroplasty: results in primary degenerative arthritis of the elbow. Clin Orthop Relat Res 2004;420:190–3.

17. Phillips NJ, Ali A, Stanley D. Treatment of primary degenerative arthritis of the elbow by ulnohumeral arthroplasty. A long-term follow-up. J Bone Joint Surg Br 2003;85(3):347–50.

18. Allen DM, Devries JP, Nunley JA. Ulnohumeral arthroplasty. Iowa Orthop J 2004;24:49–52.

19. Vingerhoeds B, Degreef I, De Smet L. Debridement arthroplasty for osteoarthritis of the elbow (Outerbridge-Kashiwagi procedure). Acta Orthop Belg 2004;70(4):306–10.

20. Kashigawi D, editor. Osteoarthritis of the elbow joint. Amersterdam: Elsevier Science Publishers; 1986. p. 177–88.

21. Wada T, Isogai S, Ishii S, et al. Debridement arthroplasty for primary osteoarthritis of the elbow. J Bone Joint Surg Am 2004;86(2):233–41.

22. O'Driscoll SW. Operative treatment of elbow arthritis. Curr Opin Rheumatol 1995;7(2):103–6.

23. Ogilvie-Harris DJ, Gordon R, MacKay M. Arthroscopic treatment for posterior impingement in degenerative arthritis of the elbow. Arthroscopy 1995;11(4): 437–43.

24. Steinmann SP, King GJ, Savoie FH 3rd. Arthroscopic treatment of the arthritic elbow. J Bone Joint Surg Am 2005;87(9):2114–21.

25. Gramstad GD, Galatz LM. Management of elbow osteoarthritis. J Bone Joint Surg Am 2006;88(2):421–30.

26. Steinmann SP, King GJ, Savoie FH 3rd. Arthroscopic treatment of the arthritic elbow. Instr Course Lect 2006;55:109–17.

27. Adams JE, Steinmann SP. The stiff elbow: degenerative joint disease. In: Savoie FH, Field LD, editors. AANA advanced arthroscopy: the wrist and elbow. Philadelphia: Saunders/Elsevier; 2010. p. 63–70.

Arthrodesis of the Elbow

Lee M. Reichel, MD[a,b], Brett P. Wiater, MD[c],
Jeffery Friedrich, MD[d], Douglas P. Hanel, MD[e,*]

KEYWORDS

- Elbow fusion • Elbow arthrodesis • Elbow salvage
- Failed elbow

ARTHRODESIS OF THE ELBOW: INDICATIONS

Elbow arthrodesis (EA) is the most disabling arthrodesis that can be performed in the upper extremity. Once the elbow is in a fixed position, the remaining joints in the extremity are unable to compensate for the loss of motion. EA should only be performed when other motion-preserving interventions are not possible. Total elbow arthroplasty is reserved for functionally older patients without significant weight-bearing demands. Proposed indications for EA include chronic infection, acute traumatic nonreconstructible elbow injuries in the functionally young, posttraumatic arthritis or instability in the functionally young, and failed total elbow arthroplasty. The goal of EA should be to relieve pain and to retain function that would be lost with amputation. When planning for EA, the surgeon must have an understanding of how to approach elbow arthrodesis in the setting of acute and late reconstructive elbow trauma and to be able to anticipate and manage potential complications. Realistic patient expectations are paramount.

LITERATURE REVIEW

EA is seldom performed and the literature reflects this, consisting of case reports and small case series. Despite the lack of higher levels of evidence, the advice in these case series cannot be overstated. The available literature represents decades of surgeon trial and error with respect to patient selection, surgical technique, and avoidance of complications (**Table 1**). Early reports focused on EA in the setting of tuberculosis.[1–4] It was recognized in these early cases that obtaining solid fusion of an elbow is a difficult task. Nickerson stated in 1942, "...that ankylosing operations for tuberculosis of the elbow in adults have been disappointing in their end results insofar as obtaining fusion is concerned."[2] Early techniques involved placing bone grafts around the elbow without internal fixation and were followed by prolonged immobilization.[2,4–7]

Nickerson[2] described placing a wedge of olecranon against the posterior humerus and was able to achieve acceptable outcomes. In describing a 49-year-old man who underwent EA for tuberculosis he states, "The elbow is clinically fused. He does a good day's work as a farm hand and suffers no pain whatever. All the sinuses are closed. Pronation and supination in the forearm is about 40% of normal."[2]

In a later report, Van Gorder in 1959 described a "central-graft" operation for elbow fusion.[4,8] In

The authors have nothing to disclose.
a University of Washington, Seattle, WA, USA
b Department of Orthopedic Surgery, Baylor College of Medicine, Ben Taub General Hospital, 1504 Taub Loop, 5B, Houston, TX 77030, USA
c Department of Orthopaedics and Sports Medicine, University of Washington, 1959 North East Pacific Street, Seattle, WA 98195, USA
d Plastics and Reconstructive Surgery, Department of Surgery, University of Washington, 1959 North East Pacific Street, Seattle, WA 98195, USA
e Department of Orthopaedics and Sports Medicine, Harborview Medical Center, University of Washington, 325 Ninth Avenue, Box 359798, Seattle, WA 98195, USA
* Corresponding author.
E-mail address: dhanel@uw.edu

Hand Clin 27 (2011) 179–186
doi:10.1016/j.hcl.2011.02.002
0749-0712/11/$ – see front matter © 2011 Published by Elsevier Inc.

Table 1
Important contributions made by selected authors to our understanding of the principles of elbow arthrodesis

Important Contributions	Year	Surgical Pearls
Wittek[22]	1914	First report of elbow arthrodesis
Steindler[5]	1923	Bone graft
Muller et al[13]	1969	Compression at fusion site
Spier[23]	1973	Plate and screw internal fixation
Arafiles[24]	1981	Recommend excision of radial head
RashKoff and Burkhalter[25]	1986	Anterior or posterior plate fusion
McAuliffe et al[11]	1992	When compression plating, bring the plate past any prior pin sites to avoid periprosthetic fracture
McAuliffe et al[11]	1992	Open wound healing possible
Presnel and Chillag[26]	1995	Radial humeral fusion technique described when ulna deficient
Ring et al[14]	1999	Vascularized fibular graft when massive bone loss

this operation, the "Hatt bayonet osteotome is driven up through the olecranon into the humerus and large rectangular bone graft obtained from the tibia or fibula is driven up in the hole."[4] Patients were then immobilized for 3 to 4 months in a shoulder spica plaster cast.[4] Of the 6 elbow central graft fusions he performed, 2 of the bone grafts fractured and were revised and using a stainless steel plate and screws. Van Gorder and Chen[4] concluded, "the experience has not been a happy one, and the opportunity to see any good results from this operation in tuberculosis elbows has not occurred. At the present time, with the use of anti-tuberculosis drugs, it is hoped that surgery may no longer be necessary in the treatment of tuberculosis of the elbow."[4]

Later series described new techniques for elbow arthrodesis based on advancements in internal fixation, external fixation, and microsurgery.[4,6,9–12] In 1969, Muller and colleagues[13] and the AO (Arbeitsgemeinschaft Für Osteosynthesefragen) group recommending applying compression between the distal humerus and olecranon by use of hardware. A partially threaded cancellous screw

and washer fixed the olecranon to the humerus and was augmented with an external fixator compression device. Although this was only a case study, multiple reports that followed demonstrated improved fusion rates when compared with the noncompression techniques. For example, Koch and Lipscomb[9], Steindler[5], Hallock[1], Staples[6], and Brittain[7] achieved a 47% successful arthrodesis rate using wires, pins and plaster. In contrast, Rashkoff and colleagues[25] achieved a 100% rate fusion in 6 patients using anterior or posterior compression plating. In 1981, Ring and colleagues[14] reported on the use of vascularized fibular graft for bony defects about the elbow; in one case, the defect included the elbow joint and a successful elbow arthrodesis was obtained (**Box 1**).

There is limited data regarding functional outcomes following elbow arthrodesis. Only 3 published series with greater than 10 subjects were identified in the English language literature.[9,11,15] Koch and Lipscomb[9] described the Mayo Clinic experience of elbow arthrodesis in 17 subjects during the years 1921 to 1962. In this series, a 47% fusion rate was reported. The investigators recognized that compression in general was beneficial in fusion operations but were hesitant to support using compression for elbow arthrodesis because they had no experience with it. McAuliffe and colleagues[11] and Koller and colleagues[16] described a case series of elbow fusions using compression internal and external fixation techniques. Fifteen subjects underwent EA using compression plating primarily for open, infected, high-energy injuries with associated bone loss. The investigators reported a 93% successful fusion rate with no fixation failures. Two subjects required revision scar operations and 2 sustained postoperative forearm fractures.

Koller and colleagues[16] reviewed 14 subjects following elbow arthrodesis. They reported 4 occurrences of skin breakdown, 3 deep infections, and 4 cases of implant failure with loss of stability

Box 1
Summary of import observations regarding surgical technique

Surgical technique recomendations

1. Debride olecranon and humerus to bleeding surfaces
2. Transpose ulnar nerve
3. Excise the radial head
4. Bulk allograft placement
5. Compression plate arthrodesis extending past any prior pin sites

and delayed union. Range of motion and functional abilities were described in 7 of these subjects. No subject with an elbow fused at greater than 100° was able to touch their mouth; forearm supination was limited to 52% and pronation to 35%.[16] Nagy and Tang[17,18] reported that all subjects with the elbow immobilized at 90° cannot bring their hand to their mouth. Both studies allude to the difficulties that a fused elbow presents to personal hygiene and activities of daily living.

Four studies have been published assessing functional elbow range of motion and compensatory joint motion that relate to optimal positioning of elbow arthrodesis. In 1981, Morrey and colleagues[19] performed a biomechanical study of normal functional elbow motion in 33 normal subjects using a triaxial electrogoniometer measuring elbow flexion-extension and pronation-supination in various activities of daily living. The conclusion was that most activities of daily living can be accomplished with a flexion arch of 100° (30–130) and 100° arch of pronation-supination (50–50).[19] They demonstrated that hand to waist required at least 100° of elbow flexion and hand to any part of the body above the waist required 120° or greater.[19] This study related the position of elbow flexion to functional activities and demonstrates that greater than 100° of elbow flexion are needed for many activities of daily living. Although providing a useful description of functional elbow motion, Morrey did not provide specific recommendations of the optimal position for elbow arthrodesis.

Two reports specifically designed to assess optimal positioning for elbow arthrodesis followed Morrey's report. The first by Nagy and colleagues[18] in 1999 simulated elbow arthrodesis in 25 volunteers by immobilizing them in 45° or 90° of elbow flexion for 24 hours and having each subject rate their abilities to perform various tasks. A total of 22 of 25 subjects favored 90° of flexion as their preferred position when asked to choose a preference for positioning during activities of daily living. Three subjects preferred 45° as their position of arthrodesis. Two of these three subjects had performed the trial immobilization during work. These investigators suggested that a more extended position of elbow arthrodesis may be preferred depending on the type of work performed by the patient.[18]

The second report examining the optimal position of EA was performed by Tang and colleagues[17] in 2001. Twenty-four healthy subjects were placed in a locked hinged elbow brace at 20° increments from 30° to 130°. Personal care, hygiene, and activities of daily living were assessed. Functional scores improved for personal care hygiene tasks and activities of daily living at increasing levels of elbow flexion peaking at 110°. When comparing functional scores at the 90° position verses the 110° they demonstrated a significant advantage to the 110° position. An admitted concern in their study design was that the study tasks primarily involved those upper extremity activities that required greater amounts of elbow flexion, biasing higher scoring by participants of the 110 degree position.

In 1992, O'Neill and colleagues[20] performed the only study specifically designed to assess compensatory motion of the shoulder and wrist. In this series, 10 subjects completed tasks indicative of normal elbow motion and then repeated these tasks while wearing a brace immobilizing their elbow at 50°, 70°, 90°, and 110°. A 3 Space Isotrak system (Polhemus Navigation Sciences Division, McDonnell Douglas Electronics, Colchester, VT, USA) was used to measure their shoulder motion and a triaxial goniometer was used to measure wrist motion. The conclusion was that, "that the primary function of the shoulder complex and the elbow are mutually exclusive therefore minimal compensatory motion occurs at the shoulder complex after elbow arthrodesis." In addition they noted, "that there is not a single optimal elbow position for all activities."[20]

In addition, the position of the elbow affects grip and key pinch strength. Mathiowetz and colleagues[21] tested 29 female occupational therapy students using a Jamar dynamometer (Item 3363; G.E. Miller, Inc, Yonkers, NY, USA) and found that bilateral grip strength and dominant-hand key pinch strength were significantly increased with the elbow flexed at 90° when compared with full elbow extension.

THE AUTHORS' EXPERIENCE
Surgical Technique

Preoperative planning involves a thorough examination of the extremity, including documentation of vascular status and neurologic function. Baseline motor strength is recorded as well as 2-point discrimination sensibility.

Previous incisions, in chronic cases, and the extent of soft-tissue damage, in acute cases, are noted.

Positioning

The quality of the soft-tissue cover directs patient positioning. If the soft-tissue envelope is intact, the operation is performed with patients supine and the involved extremity resting on an arm board. The advantages of supine positioning include the ability to operate on the full circumference of the elbow with relative ease and the ease with which intraoperative fluoroscopic imaging can be obtained. If there is a large soft-tissue defect that cannot be covered with local flaps, the procedure is performed in a lateral decubitus position. The injured extremity, the ipsilateral thorax, and ipsilateral thigh are prepped into the operative field. The injured extremity is placed over a well-padded adjustable arm rail. The exposed thorax provides access to the ipsilateral latissimus dorsi. This muscle may be used for soft-tissue coverage at the end of the case. The exposed thigh serves as a potential donor site for split-thickness skin graft.

The procedure is performed under a general anesthetic. Tourniquets are not used.

The planned incisions are infused with 0.25% bupivacaine combined with 1:100,000 dilute epinephrine. When possible, a straight posterior incision is used. This incision starts at the junction of the proximal and mid one-third of the arm, is directed lateral to the tip of the olecranon, and ends along the posterolateral border of the ulna, half way down the forearm. If operating through a prior incision, it may be necessary to extend the incisions further distally and proximally to mobilize soft tissues. Full-thickness skin flaps are elevated. Attention is directed first at isolating and protecting neurovascular structures. If a medially based incision is made, the ulnar nerve is identified and preserved. Special care is taken to follow the ulnar nerve from proximal to distal, especially when there is a history of previous surgery. When dissecting through a previously operated and scarred field, the incision is extended proximally until a plane of normal tissue is identified. The medial intermuscular septum is removed. Osborne's ligament and the fascial bands of the flexor carpi ulnaris are divided and the origin of the flexor-pronator mass are elevated from the distal humerus. The dissection is continued along the volar surface of the brachialis and directed laterally until the median nerve and the brachial artery are identified and protected. The ulnar nerve is transposed anteriorly. With the medial structures protected, the lateral skin flap is elevated. Upon reaching the lateral edge of triceps muscle, small perforator vessels can be seen running within the lateral intermuscular septum. These vessels are branches of the profunda brachii artery, the artery that accompanies the radial nerve through the spiral groove as it passes from the posterior to anterior arm. Using these branches as landmarks, one can easily identify and protect the radial nerve.

When the elbow joint is approached laterally, the triceps muscle insertion and anconeus are kept in continuity and peeled off the proximal ulna and olecranon.

The elbow joint is now exposed. Joint exposure may be dictated by a traumatic arthrotomy or, in elective cases, is made on the most mobile side of the joint. In either case, the collateral ligaments, anterior and posterior joint capsule, synovium, and loose osteocartilaginous structures are removed. The remaining articular surfaces are denuded of cartilage until subchondral cancellous bone is exposed. The interface between the distal humerus and the olecranon are prepared and provisional fixation secures the elbow in its predetermined position of the fusion. The radiocapitellar joint is left intact if excessive resection of the trochlear is not required and the articular surfaces of the capitellum and radial head are in good condition.

Definitive fixation is secured with an 18- or 20-hole 3.5-mm low contact dynamic compression plate bent midway and placed over the posterior distal humerus and proximal ulna. If there is inadequate bone stock, then a femoral condyle allograft may be useful. The plate is secured to the bone with 3.5-mm cortical screws of appropriate length. Allograft is placed about the fusion site. Wound drains are placed and the wounds are closed in layers. A compression dressing is applied and the limb is initially immobilized on pillows and a sling later. Drains are removed when there output is less than 30 mL in a 24-hour period. Shoulder, forearm, wrist, and digit motion are started on the first days postoperatively but stresses upon the elbow are avoided until there is radiographic evidence of boney union.

If, in the setting of trauma, the wound cannot be closed with local tissue and the extent of the deficit would require more than 1 week of negative pressure dressings, then the ipsilateral latissimus dorsi muscle is harvested as a pedicle or free flap, inset about the defect, and skin grafted primarily. Postoperative management in this setting is altered to protect the flap and skin grafts.

THE AUTHORS' EXPERIENCE

From 2004 to 2009 the senior author performed 12 elbow arthrodesis procedures at Harborview Medical Center. All patients were followed to radiographic union and wound healing, except for a single patient with an infected nonunion of his elbow arthrodesis who left the country and was thus lost to follow-up. The average length of follow-up was 39 months.

All patients were men and the mean age was 39 years. Eight cases were originally open elbow fractures that then developed posttraumatic arthritis. Six of these were in patients who sustained open distal humerus fractures with significant bone and joint defects. Two of these patients had associated olecranon fractures. The remaining 2 open injuries represented an open Monteggia fracture and a patient with combined open proximal radius and ulna fractures.

A single patient presented with posttraumatic arthritis following a closed olecranon fracture sustained 17 years prior. One patient reported a closed elbow dislocation event many years prior, and the final patient had a remote history of elbow trauma but no specific elbow injury could be ascertained.

Of the 10 patients for whom the mechanism of injury was known, 4 were the result of high-energy, high-speed automobile accidents, 2 were secondary to motorcycle accidents, 3 resulted from a fall from a height, and 1 was secondary to a gun shot.

Four patients underwent elbow arthrodesis within 5 months or less of their original injury. Four others underwent elbow arthrodesis at greater than 8 years after their original injuries. One patient underwent elbow fusion during his initial hospital admission. Five of the 12 patients required flap coverage.

Ten of 12 patients (83%) required secondary procedures. A total of 19 secondary procedures were performed in these 10 patients resulting in an average of 1.6 secondary procedures per patient. Secondary procedures included incision and debridements for infection, hardware removal for symptomatic hardware, medial epicondylectomy for skin breakdown over a bony prominence, pedicle or free-flap soft-tissue coverage, and 1 patient underwent a resection arthroplasty. Five of 12 patients underwent repeat bone grafting for delayed or nonunion, with a delayed union or nonunion rate of 42%. There was hardware failure in 1 patient in whom 2 screws used for fixation of a free fibula graft to augment his elbow arthrodesis. This fixation was revised to a compression plate.

Four elbow arthrodesis developed infections, yielding an overall infection rate of 33%. Two patients developed infected nonunions. Both of these patients had histories of prior open fractures. One patient developed an infection in the setting of a bulk allograft used for his elbow arthrodesis; the infection cleared following removal of the allograft. The fourth patient with an infection had previously undergone attempted elbow arthrodesis by another surgeon and presented with a septic nonunion. With revision surgery and implant removal, arthrodesis was successful and infection was suppressed. At final follow-up all infections were resolved or suppressed except for 1 patient with an infected nonunion who was lost to follow-up.

There were no cases of major nerve injury associated with the procedure.

Seven of 12 patients completed a questionnaire rating their pain as none, mild, moderate, severe, or extreme. On average, pain was reported between mild and moderate. Seven of 12 patients reported they felt less capable, confident, or useful because of their arm, shoulder, or hand. Seven of 12 patients also noted that their extremity interfered with their normal social activities (**Box 2**).

CASE EXAMPLE

A 19-year-old farm worker presented to Harborview Medical Center after sustaining injuries in a high-speed automobile accident. The radiograph in **Fig. 1** demonstrates the position of the distal humerus in the emergency room. After stabilization of concomitant systemic injuries, his upper-extremity wound was debrided, a negative-pressure dressing applied, and his elbow stabilized with an external fixator (**Fig. 2**). At time of the injury, the distal one-half of the humerus was stripped of all soft tissues and the distal humerus was devoid of any viable articular cartilage (**Fig. 3**). The major peripheral nerves and vessels were in continuity; however, clinical examination revealed no radial and ulnar motor function. An elbow arthrodesis was recommended.

A free vascularized fibular graft was used to reconstruct the massive humeral bone loss (**Figs. 4** and **5**). Fixation consisted of screws placed through the proximal and distal bony interfaces augmented with an external fixator (**Figs. 6** and **7**). The external fixator was removed 4 months later, when radiographic evidence of osteosynthesis was noted. At 3 months after surgery, ulnar and radial motor function returned. At 1 year following the accident, the patient returned after developing a dull nagging pain about the elbow. Radiographs revealed broken screws and a hypertrophic nonunion of the distal graft and olecranon (**Fig. 8**). Revision arthrodesis with a compression plate and bone grafting led to successful union and return to work as a farm hand (**Fig. 9**).

Box 2
Summary of expected postoperative outcomes

Expectations of outcomes

1. Postoperative major nerve dysfunction rare
2. Revision bone grafting probable
3. Unanticipated hardware and bony irritation probable
4. Infection likely to resolve with antibiotics and union
5. Patient satisfaction tempered by functional loss

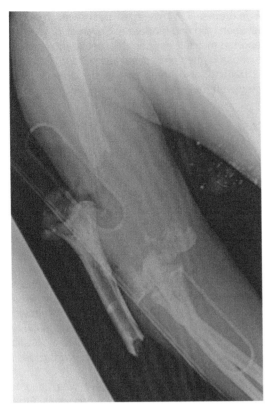

Fig. 1. The patient presented to the emergency room with a devastating open humerus fracture.

DISCUSSION

Elbow arthrodesis is an uncommon procedure that should be performed when there are no other reasonable reconstructive options. The indications for surgery include infection, nonreconstructible acute trauma, failed total elbow arthroplasty, and posttraumatic arthritis in patients who are functionally too young to undergo arthroplasty.

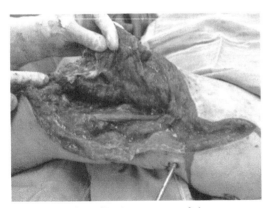

Fig. 2. The devitalized segment of humerus was removed. The radial nerve is visualized as intact within the wound. A large triceps laceration is present.

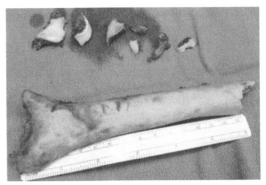

Fig. 3. Devitalized segment of humerus with comminuted nonreconstructible distal humerus fragments.

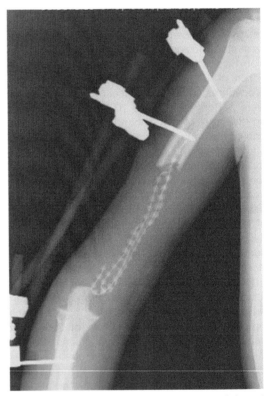

Fig. 4. Radiograph following debridement of devitalized humerus and placement of antibiotic beads demonstrated massive bone loss.

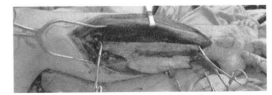

Fig. 5. Harvest of free fibular graft to bridge humeral defect for extremity reconstruction with elbow fusion.

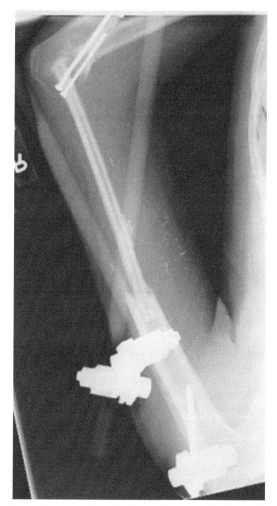

Fig. 6. Postoperative fixation of the free fibular graft.

In the posttraumatic setting, the surgeon must be prepared to deal with a poor soft-tissue envelope, previous hardware placement, scarred tissue beds, nerves encased in scar or bone, and altered bony anatomy.

Technical considerations include the method of fusion and positioning of the elbow. The authors

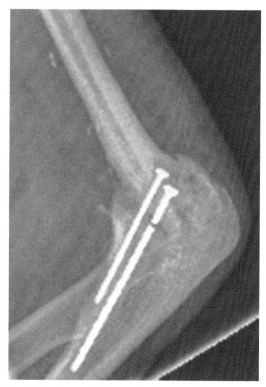

Fig. 8. Hardware failure and hypertrophic nonunion of elbow arthrodesis.

think that, when possible, compression plating is superior to other methods of fixation and agree with McAuliffe and colleagues[11] that it provides improved rigidity without the need for external fixation. As delineated by O'Neill and colleagues[20] there is no optimal position for elbow arthrodesis and at every position some function will be lost. Published functional studies infer that an optimal position likely lies somewhere between 90° and 110° for so-called intraperson activities.[17–19] However, it has been suggested that extraperson activities may be better served with fusion in

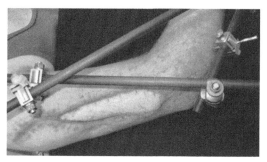

Fig. 7. Postoperative wound healing of osteocutaneous free fibula flap.

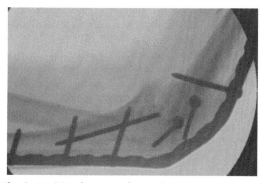

Fig. 9. Revision bone grafting of elbow hypertrophic nonunion with addition of compression plate.

greater degrees of extension. In the elective setting, the least debilitating position for patients can be determined after discussing needs and desires and, if mobility allows, splinting the limb in varying positions. Patients then determine the least burdensome position by trial. In the acute trauma setting, the authors aim for fusion at a position between 90° and 100°.

As other authors have suggested, this salvage procedure has a high complication rate and frequently requires secondary procedures.[11] Patients should be counseled that postoperative complications are to be expected and the need for further surgery is the rule rather than the exception. Complications include infection, delayed union or nonunion requiring bone grafting, revision internal fixation, hardware or bony prominence irritation requiring removal or osteoplasty, and periprosthetic fracture. These complications are similar to that reported in other series.[11]

Since it was first described in 1914 by Wittek,[22] EA continues to be a challenging undertaking with a high incidence of complications and resulting in significant functional disability. The optimal position of elbow arthrodesis remains unclear. For the most part, this is a procedure of last resort and should only be performed when no other options for limb salvage exist.

REFERENCES

1. Hallock H. Fusion of the elbow joint for tuberculosis: a new technique and a report of three cases. J Bone Joint Surg Am 1932;14:1–10.
2. Nickerson SH. A modified approach in surgery for tuberculosis of the elbow in the adult. Am J Surg 1942;56:483–7.
3. Gellman M. Arthrodesis of the elbow a preliminary report of a new operation. J Bone Joint Surg Am 1947;29(4):850–2.
4. Van Gorder GW, Chen CM. The central-graft operation for fusion of tuberculous knees, ankles, and elbows. J Bone Joint Surg Am 1959;41:1029–46.
5. Steindler A. Reconstructive surgery of the upper extremity. New York: Appleton; 1923. p. 23–9.
6. Staples OS. Arthrodesis of the elbow joint. J Bone Joint Surg Am 1952;34(1):207–10.
7. Brittian H. Architectural principles in arthrodesis. Edinburgh (UK): E&S Livingstone; 1942.
8. Hatt RN. The central bone graft in joint arthrodesis. J Bone Joint Surg 1940;22:393–402.
9. Koch M, Lipscomb PR. Arthrodesis of the elbow. Clin Orthop Relat Res 1967;50:151–7.
10. Weiland AJ, Kleinert HE, Kutz JE, et al. Free vascularized bone grafts in surgery of the upper extremity. J Hand Surg 1979;4(2):129–44.
11. McAuliffe JA, Burkhalter WE, Ouellette EA, et al. Compression plate arthrodesis of the elbow. J Bone Joint Surg Br 1992;74(2):300–4.
12. Lerner A, Stein H, Calif E. Unilateral hinged external fixation frame for elbow compression arthrodesis: the stepwise attainment of a stable 90-degree flexion position: a case report. J Orthop Trauma 2005;19(1):52–5.
13. Muller ME, Allgower M, Willenegger H. Manual der osteosynthese. Berlin-Heidelberg (Germany): Springer; 1969. New York [in German].
14. Ring D, Jupiter JB, Toh S. Transarticular bony defects after trauma and sepsis: arthrodesis using vascularized fibular transfer. Plast Reconstr Surg 1999;104(2):426–34.
15. Bilic R, Kolundzic R, Bicanic G, et al. Elbow arthrodesis and its alternatives. Orthopade 1996;25(2):112–20 [in German].
16. Koller H, Kolb K, Assuncao A, et al. The fate of elbow arthrodesis: indications, techniques, and outcome in fourteen patients. J Shoulder Elbow Surg 2008;17(2):293–306.
17. Tang C, Roidis N, Itamura J, et al. The effect of simulated elbow arthrodesis on the ability to perform activities of daily living. J Hand Surg Am 2001;26(6):1146–50.
18. Nagy SM, Szabo RM, Sharkey NA. Unilateral elbow arthrodesis: the preferred position. J South Orthop Assoc 1999;8(2):80–5.
19. Morrey BF, Askew LJ, Chao EY. A biomechanical study of normal functional elbow motion. J Bone Joint Surg Am 1981;63(6):872–7.
20. O'Neill OR, Morrey BF, Tanaka S, et al. Compensatory motion in the upper extremity after elbow arthrodesis. Clin Orthop Relat Res 1992;(281):89–96.
21. Mathiowetz V, Rennells C, Donahoe L. Effect of elbow position on grip and key pinch strength. J Hand Surg 1985;10(5):694–7.
22. Wittek A. Verh Dtsch Orthop Ges XIII Congress 1914;9 [in German].
23. Spier W. [Compression arthrodesis of the elbow joint]. Monatsschr Unfallheilkd Versicher Versorg Verkehrsmed 1973;76(6):274–7 [in German].
24. Arafiles RP. A new technique of fusion for tuberculous arthritis of the elbow. J Bone Joint Surg Am 1981;63(9):1396–400.
25. Rashkoff E, Burkhalter WE. Arthrodesis of the salvage elbow. Orthopedics 1986;9(5):733–8.
26. Presnal BP, Chillag KJ. Radiohumeral arthrodesis for salvage of failed total elbow arthroplasty. J Arthroplasty 1995;10(5):699–701.

Elbow Interposition Arthroplasty

Darwin D. Chen, MD, David A. Forsh, MD,
Michael R. Hausman, MD*

KEYWORDS

- Elbow arthritis • Interposition arthroplasty
- Upper extremity surgery

Loss of motion and pain secondary to elbow arthritis is one of the most challenging problems affecting the upper extremity. Painful elbow arthrosis, either primary or posttraumatic, in high-demand and younger patients remains a difficult clinical scenario. Longevity concerns and limitations on function and weight bearing may preclude total elbow arthroplasty in this population, because a failed prosthetic elbow may have no satisfactory salvage option, particularly if the cause of failure is sepsis. Therefore, interposition arthroplasty may be a more conservative and appropriate treatment. Although pain relief and restoration of motion are not as good as with a prosthetic elbow replacement, there are no functional limitations after interposition arthroplasty. Furthermore, interposition arthroplasty preserves the bony architecture of the elbow and can be revised to a total elbow arthroplasty, if necessary, at a later date.

HISTORICAL PERSPECTIVE

Elbow arthritis, and its associated pain and loss of motion, is a serious condition that profoundly affects function and quality of life. It is frequently associated with elbow trauma, overuse injury, or rheumatoid arthritis, and thus tends to affect a younger patient population.[1] Basic activities of daily living, such as grooming, feeding, and personal hygiene, require a 30° to 130° arc of motion, according to Morrey.[2] Osteoarthritis, affecting an older patient population, is characterized by peripheral osteophytes causing pain at terminal flexion and extension and limitation of motion. However, the central portion of the joint is preserved and CT scan demonstrates a normal central articular surface rimmed by hypertrophic osteophytes. Debridement of the joint, either by open means, such as the Outerbridge-Kashiwagi type procedure, or arthroscopically, are satisfying solutions to patients and surgeon alike, providing long-term relief of pain and improvement in motion.[3]

However, in contrast to this group, primary arthritis, rheumatoid disease, and posttraumatic arthritis are characterized by unrelenting pain throughout the limited arc of motion and radiographic studies demonstrate pan-articular joint destruction with loss of cartilage and narrowing of the entire joint space. In such patients, debridement alone will not alleviate the pain or improve the motion, and some form of arthroplasty is required. Although semiconstrained total elbow arthroplasty (STEA) has had good early results, longevity and concerns with revision and infection limit its use in younger, more active patients.[4–6]

Functional limitations restricting patients to lifting no more than 5 kg are advised after STEA.[6] Joint replacement is generally not recommended for posttraumatic dysfunction primarily because affected patients are usually aged less than 60 years and may have unsatisfactory long-term results.[1] Resection arthroplasty, resulting in a flail, unstable joint, is an unsatisfactory procedure with extremely limited function and is not an attractive option in younger patients. External bracing cannot substitute for a stable joint. Similarly, arthrodesis is poorly tolerated. The final alternative is interposition

The authors have nothing to disclose.

Department of Orthopaedic Surgery, Mount Sinai School of Medicine, 5 East 98th Street, 9th Floor, New York, NY 10029, USA

* Corresponding author.

E-mail address: Michael.Hausman@mountsinai.org

Hand Clin 27 (2011) 187–197

doi:10.1016/j.hcl.2011.01.002

arthroplasty, an old operation that has been variously modified by the use of an interposition membrane of fascia or dermis and distraction with an articulated external fixator.[7]

Interposition arthroplasty has been performed on many joints, including the hip and temporomandibular joints, and is considered a preprosthetic alternative for younger patients. It was reported by Verneuil as early as 1860 and again in 1924 by Campbell.[8,9] The addition of hinged distraction is new and was first described by Volkov and Oganesian[7] in 1975 and Deland and colleagues[10] in 1983. Bony anatomy is maintained and ligaments are preserved, repaired, or reconstructed because stability is required for a good result. Long-term outcome data is available from the rheumatoid population with durable and satisfactory results reported. Ljung and colleagues[11] demonstrated 6-year follow-up with 21 of 28 elbows having no pain or slight pain with motion. A total of 22 of these elbows had similar results at rest. Fernandez-Palazzi and colleagues[12] reported 20-year follow-up results of interposition arthroplasty in children and adolescents with 5 of 12 elbows showing good-to-excellent results. Although pain relief and motion are not as good as STEA, durability may be better and revision to STEA is possible because bone stock is preserved.

The presence of normal bone anatomy as an absolute prerequisite for successful interposition arthroplasty has been repeatedly demonstrated. Kita[13] reported 31 subjects with fascia lata interposition without distraction. The 19-year follow-up showed prolonged pain relief and best results with patients with rheumatoid arthritis. All poor outcomes were associated with instability. A 14-year follow-up by Knight and Van Zandt[14] of 45 cases revealed 50% of subjects with good results and a 20% failure rate associated with instability. Most recently, Nolla and colleagues[15] reported their results of 13 severe posttraumatic elbow arthrosis treated with interposition arthroplasty and temporary hinged external fixation. Two elbows were considered to have failed because of early postoperative instability and their results were classified as poor. They had 4 subjects with severe instability associated with bone loss of the distal humerus or trochlear notch. Prior series of interposition arthroplasty as reported by Fox and colleagues[16] as well as Cheng and Morrey[17] emphasized the importance of stability as a determinant of outcome.

INDICATIONS

Interposition arthroplasty is a salvage procedure with limited indications for the painful and stiff arthritic elbow and is best indicated for severe posttraumatic elbow arthritis or stage II or IIA rheumatoid arthritis in young, high-demand patients with near normal bone anatomy (**Figs. 1** and **2**).[18] As previously described, adequate bone stock and no gross instability are imperative for successful outcomes in posttraumatic and rheumatoid elbows. Although ligament insufficiency in and of itself is not a contraindication, because both medial and lateral collateral ligaments may be reconstructed with grafts, instability caused by loss of bone stock is a contraindication, unless the bone loss is corrected by vascularized or successful nonvascularized bone grafting before performing the arthroplasty.

Wright and colleagues[19] have defined the presence of active infection, open physes, and absence of flexor motor power as contraindications for interposition arthroplasty. Patients aged more than 60 years who place lower demands on their severely arthritic elbows are not contraindicated but might be better served with STEA.[20–22]

TECHNIQUE

Patients are placed in either the supine or lateral decubitus position. The authors use an articulated shoulder positioner attached to the forearm, to help suspend the forearm over the chest, permitting the operation to be performed in the supine position (**Fig. 3**). A regional anesthetic is administered via an indwelling axillary or intrascalene catheter. A sterile tourniquet is applied. There are 2 general approaches described for interposition arthroplasty: the medial-lateral and the posterior approaches. Although the Mayo-modified extended posterolateral approach is a good option and is commonly used for joint exposure, a posteromedial approach may be preferable for protecting the ulnar nerve and reconstructing the medial collateral ligament (MCL).

A posterior incision is made over the midline of the triceps and is extended distally in a longitudinal fashion over the olecranon and ulnar crest. The incision should be sufficiently long to expose the medial and lateral aspects of the joint easily without tension on the skin and a longer incision is preferable to more pulling with retractors. A straight incision, rather than curving around the olecranon, will result in fewer wound issues. Thick flaps should be raised between the triceps/forearm muscle fascia and subcutaneous tissue (**Fig. 4**). The ulnar nerve is identified medially and is released from the cubital tunnel. It should be freed proximally at the arcade of Struthers and distally into the flexor carpi ulnaris (**Fig. 5**), but it does not have to be fully and

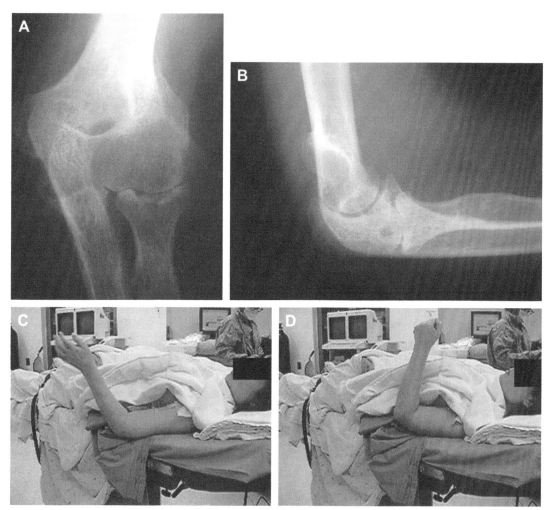

Fig. 1. (A, B) Anteroposterior and lateral radiographs of a 29-year-old patient with rheumatoid arthritis. The elbow is classified as a Mayo stage II, with loss of joint space, but relative preservation of bony architecture. (C, D) The patient has pain and a severe functional deficit because she cannot reach her mouth or head.

circumferentially mobilized if care is exercised during the procedure. The medial intermuscular septum is dissected free and excised.

The medial epicondyle is exposed. The flexor/pronator attachment and medial collateral ligament can be released in 2 different ways. They can be either dissected off subperiosteally, forming a distally based flap, or released by performing an osteotomy of the medial epicondyle (**Fig. 6**). It is important to recognize that the anterior band of the medial collateral ligament attaches onto the anterior inferior aspect of the medial epicondyle. The posterior band attaches onto the posterior inferior aspect of the medial epicondyle and forms the floor of the cubital tunnel. If a medial epicondyle osteotomy is performed, it must be deep and proximal enough to include the medial collateral ligament and the pronator attachments, respectively.

The anterior capsule is separated from the brachialis muscle and is released. Posteriorly, the triceps muscle is reflected away from the posterior capsule, and this capsule is released as well. A thorough and complete release must be performed. An attempt to hinge the joint open is made and, if exposure is adequate, the lateral collateral ligament can be spared. If exposure is inadequate, the lateral collateral ligament and extensor attachments are released subperiosteally from the lateral epicondyle. It is often possible to perform these lateral releases from the medial side with the joint hinged open. Alternatively, the Kocher interval between the anconeus and extensor carpi ulnaris can be opened from superficial to deep, releasing the extensor mass and lateral collateral ligament complex subperiosteally from the lateral epicondyle. From the lateral side,

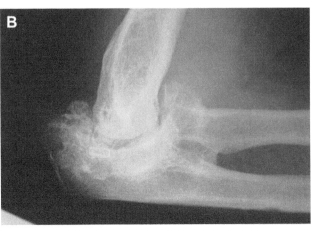

Fig. 2. (*A, B*) Anteroposterior and lateral radiographs of advanced posttraumatic elbow arthritis (note hardware from prior surgery). This patient still maintains some joint space. Interposition arthroplasty is an option only if reconstructing the MCL, and lateral ulnar collateral ligament at the time of surgery can restore stability.

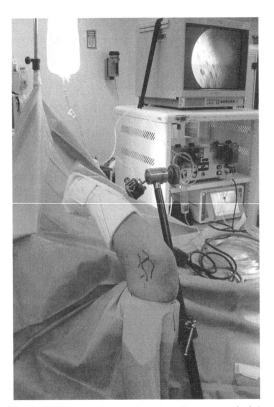

Fig. 3. Patient supine with extremity suspended in shoulder positioner.

a release of the anterior and posterior capsule from the distal humerus should also be performed.

Dislocating the elbow is the most difficult part of the operation, particularly in the stiff, posttraumatic elbow. The surgeon must be patient and sequentially extend the capsular and ligamentous release as required to dislocate the elbow. The

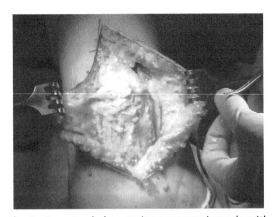

Fig. 4. An extended posterior exposure is made with thick skin flaps raised medially and laterally. The authors prefer an extended posteromedial exposure, which helps identify and protect the ulnar nerve. More important, this approach permits easy preservation of the MCL (by means of osteotomy of the medial epicondyle) or reconstruction with a graft, if necessary.

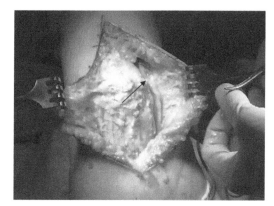

Fig. 5. Ulnar nerve unroofed proximally at the arcade of Struthers and distally into the ulnar belly of flexor carpi ulnaris (*arrow*).

amount of dissection will vary with the pathology, but will always require a thorough and complete anterior and posterior capsulectomy. In the rare case that the ulnar nerve cannot be mobilized or identified because of extensive scarring from prior surgery, it is unsafe to proceed with the dislocation of the joint because of excess traction on the nerve and high risk of neurapraxia. In this scenario, or if standard medial and lateral releases are inadequate to achieve dislocation, an olecranon osteotomy can be performed to achieve greater exposure (**Fig. 7**A, B). With the olecranon osteotomized, the triceps mass, including the posterior capsule, can be reflected with the proximal olecranon fragment, providing excellent visualization of the distal humerus for placement of the interposition graft (see **Fig. 7**C). The osteotomy can be repaired later using standard techniques, such as tension band wiring. This exposure is generally the most challenging part of the case and persistence and patience are often required.

The joint is hinged open and the articular surface of the distal humerus is evaluated. A synovectomy is performed anteriorly and posteriorly. Osteophytes are debrided with a rongeur, and any remaining cartilage on the distal humerus is removed with a large burr or a curette (**Fig. 8**). Care should be taken not to penetrate or remove subchondral bone because it is the strongest osseous portion that withstands load. Decortication increases the chance of late subsidence and one should err on the side of less debridement rather than risk injuring and resecting subchondral bone. At this point, if an articulated external fixator is to be used, the axis pin for external fixation can be placed.

The axis of the fixator must coincide with the axis of rotation of the elbow joint to prevent binding, incongruous motion, or wearing and shearing of the graft. The pin must pass through the axis of rotation of the elbow, which is approximately the center of circles defined by the circumferences of the trochlea and the capitellum. With good exposure of the distal humerus, the pin may be passed freehand (**Fig. 9**A) using a large anterior cruciate ligament drill guide, or by the radiographic method described previously.[23,24] Fluoroscopy confirms proper placement of the axis pin (see **Fig. 9**A, B).

A variety of graft materials have been described, including dermis, fascia lata, allograft fascia and allograft fascia and tendon, among others, but the authors favor either a fascia lata graft, Achilles tendon allograft, or AlloDerm (Lifecell, Branchburg, NJ, USA). The graft can be fashioned to the dimensions of the distal humerus covering areas of articular surface. Drill holes are arranged with a power-driven K-wire or drill (**Fig. 10**A). The holes need to be large enough to pass a Keith needle (see **Fig. 10**B). They should be arranged in a mattress fashion oriented proximo-distally so that elbow

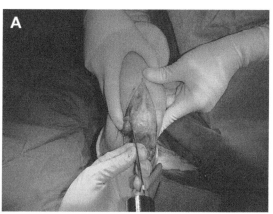

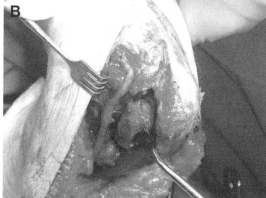

Fig. 6. (*A, B*) In this case the MCL is intact. The medial epicondyle is predrilled and osteotomized at the medial edge of the trochlea, protecting the MCL.

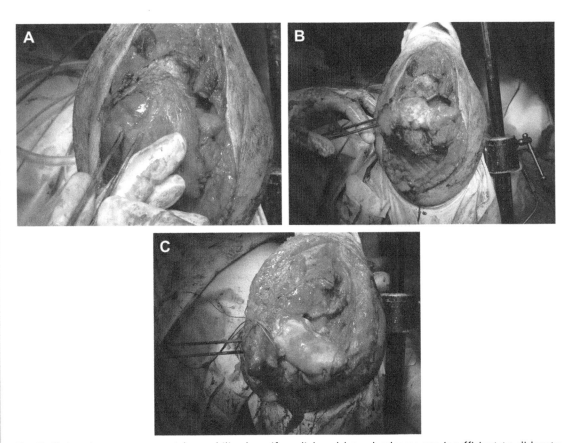

Fig. 7. If the ulnar nerve cannot be mobilized, or if medial and lateral releases are insufficient to dislocate the elbow, an olecranon osteotomy (*A, B*) can be performed to gain exposure of the distal humerus for graft placement (*C*).

flexion and extension will not tend to tear at the #2 Kevlar-reinforced sutures. Typically, 2 sets of drill holes are made just medial and lateral to the center of the articulation. Two additional sets are made

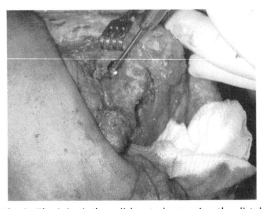

Fig. 8. The joint is then dislocated, exposing the distal humerus. The anterior and posterior capsules are released, if necessary. A rongeur, curette, or burr is used to excoriate the surface and remove any cartilage, but the humerus is not decorticated to preserve bone stock and prevent late subsidence.

over the medial and lateral-most aspects of the joint, adjacent to the condyles. Free Keith needles are used to pass braided, nonabsorbable sutures (see **Fig. 10**C, D). The graft needs to be incorporated with each pass of suture, ensuring that there is enough tension on the graft to adhere to bone. Also, if enough graft is available, it can be doubled up. Suture ends of the medial and lateral-most aspects of the joint should remain long after knot tying. They can be incorporated into the repair of the collateral ligaments. Suture anchors are another option for collateral ligament repair. Screw fixation is preferred if a medial epicondylectomy is performed.

If the medial and lateral collateral ligaments require reconstruction, this is performed before application of the external fixator. On the medial side, the technique described by Jobe and colleagues[25] is used with a palmaris tendon graft (**Fig. 11**). Laterally, options include reefing of the native capsuloligamentous complex, reconstruction with a tendon graft as described by O'Driscoll and colleagues,[26] or reconstruction with the lateral triceps tendon as described by Delamora

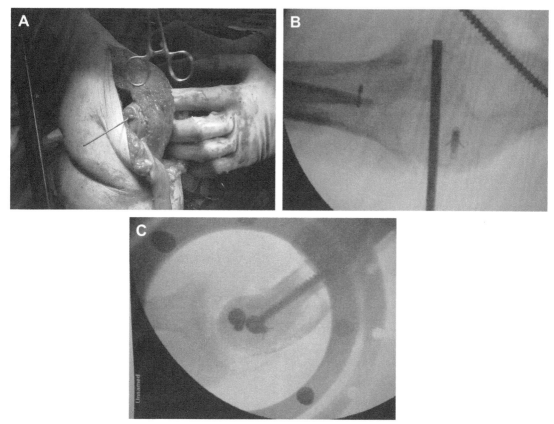

Fig. 9. (*A*) The axis pin is placed through the center of the axis of rotation of the elbow. With good exposure, this can be done freehand or with an anterior cruciate ligament-type drill guide. Correct placement of this pin is critical and its position should be confirmed by direct and radiographic inspection. (*B, C*) Anteroposterior and lateral radiographs showing correct placement of the axis.

and Hausman.[27] Alternatively, if the length of the interposition graft permits, 2 tails can be fashioned from the graft at its terminal end and used for lateral and medial collateral reconstruction as described by Larson and Morrey.[28]

Application of an articulated external fixator is also challenging and exacting. If the axis of the device does not coincide perfectly with the elbow axis of rotation, motion will be restricted and the incongruent forces will tear the graft. Interposition arthroplasty was originally described without the use of distraction and a fixator, which was added, as an innovation, by Volkov.[7–9] However, the advantages of a fixator are theoretical and have never been demonstrated. Given the difficulty of accurately reproducing the axis, the consequences of failing to do so and the added difficulty and inconvenience of postoperative management, the authors have largely abandoned the use of an external fixator in recent years.

If a fixator is to be used, the most important point in elbow external fixation is establishing congruous motion while providing distraction. Available fixators include the Morrey DJD (Stryker, Mahwah, NJ, USA), the Compass Hinge (Smith & Nephew, Memphis, TN, USA), the OptiROM Elbow Fixator (EBI, Parsippany, NJ, USA), and the Orthofix Elbow Fixator (Intavent Orthofix Ltd, Berkshire, UK). The authors prefer a fixator that permits visualization of the joint, such as the DJD, EBI, or Compass Hinge. The EBI fixator is unilateral and permits some adjustment of the axis once the humeral pins have been inserted. The Compass Hinge has a convenient clutch mechanism, allowing patients to range the elbow by simply turning a knob on the fixator. However, the axis is fixed by the first posteromedial pin inserted and cannot be adjusted. For the EBI fixator, the humeral and ulnar pins are provisionally located on the extremity with the fixator assembled. The distraction mechanism is set up to begin distraction. The 2 humeral pins are placed laterally by dissecting bluntly down to the bone to avoid injuring the radial nerve (**Fig. 12**). The axis position is confirmed once again based on the position of the fixator frame connected to the humeral and axis pins. If a circular inset guide is used and

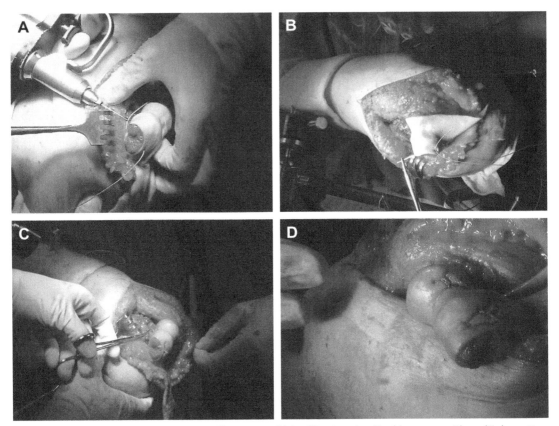

Fig. 10. (*A–D*) The membrane (in this case AlloDerm graft) is affixed to the distal humerus with multiple mattress sutures passed with a Keith needle. The graft should fit tightly and firmly.

withdrawn from the guide pin and again re-advanced, it should register perfectly. If it fails to align perfectly, adjustments should be made in the fixator frame so that there is perfect registration of the plastic axis pin insert into the EBI fixator ring.

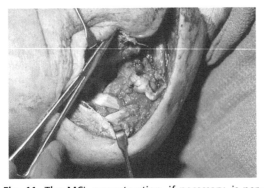

Fig. 11. The MCL reconstruction, if necessary, is performed by passing the palmaris tendon graft through the ulnar tunnel and then by passing both ends into the distal-most hole in the medial epicondyle. Both ends are secured in each tunnel and the sutures attached are tied over a bony bridge. This is referred to as the *docking procedure*.

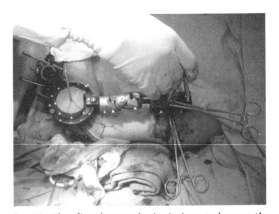

Fig. 12. The first humeral pin is inserted near the deltoid insertion. Blunt dissection protects the radial nerve. Care must be taken to avoid torqueing and shifting the axis while inserting the humeral pins. The centering guide helps to maintain the axis, but gentle technique is required. The centering guide should be lifted from the fixator after tightening the pin and fixator. It should maintain perfect registration and drop back into the fixator. Any shifting indicates that the axis has shifted and should be corrected at this point. The ulnar pins may then be inserted and the axis checked once again.

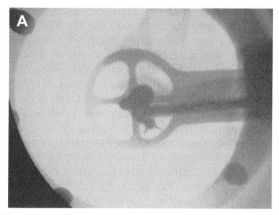
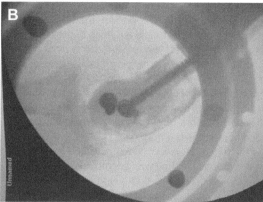

Fig. 13. (*A, B*) Distraction flexion and extension lateral radiographs.

This adjustment fixes the axis of rotation. The 2 ulnar pins are then placed. The fixator is applied and the axis pin is centered with the targeting device under fluoroscopy. After centering, the axis pin is removed and the elbow is taken through range of motion, under fluoroscopy, visualizing the ulnohumeral and the radiocapitellar articulations. Distraction should be equally distributed on anteroposterior and lateral views (**Fig. 13**). Clinically, there should be no crepitus noted throughout range of motion, and the forearm should be angled just medial to the arm in the coronal plane on full elbow flexion.

The detached muscles (flexor-pronator or common extensors) are anatomically repaired to their origins along the distal humerus. The authors' preference is to leave the ulnar nerve in situ, although other authors advocate transposition. If transposition is elected, the nerve should be widely mobilized so that it can be placed well anterior to the epicondyle rather than perched over the epicondyle. The skin is then carefully closed over a suction drain with a tight, running, subcuticular closure. One cannot be too compulsive about a careful closure because uneventful wound healing is critical to a successful outcome and the incision will be stressed and stretched early in the healing process. A light and loose dressing is applied so as not to restrict motions postoperatively and the elbow is splinted 24 to 36 hours before beginning therapy.

REHABILITATION

An indwelling axillary catheter is used for anesthesia and postoperative analgesia. Range-of-motion exercises are begun one week after surgery, with long (approximately 1 hour) cycle times, with emphasis on obtaining the maximum range of motion rather than number of cycle times. This practice is done to minimize tension and motion at the fresh incision sites, which increases inflammation, scarring, and the chance of wound healing problems. A continuous passive motion machine is not used. As healing progresses, more cycles are permitted. The rate of infusion in the

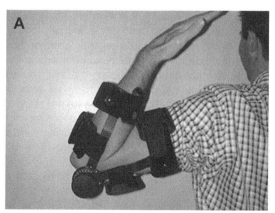
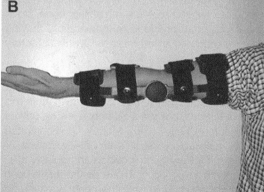

Fig. 14. Flexion (*A*) and extension (*B*) bracing.

catheter should be such as to make patients comfortable enough to perform therapy without producing total anesthesia and loss of proprioception. Care must be taken to protect the ulnar nerve from prolonged pressure, particularly during the first 24 hours when the limb may still be anesthetic and lacking protective sensation. Static progressive splinting may be used depending upon whether patients are having more difficulty in flexion or extension.

If the fixator is used, it is left in place for 8 to 12 weeks, if possible. Following removal of the fixator, the elbow undergoes static splinting for 3 to 4 months. A simple elastic bandage is used for flexion. The authors' extension splint is a simple plaster or firm plastic strip with an area cut out for the thumb. It is arc shaped to increase the rigidity. Instead of molding the splint to the patients' arm, it is made straight, which is the desired position. In this way, the arm bowstrings across the splint and there is always a corrective force. Extending the splint from the hand to the shoulder increases the moment arms acting on the elbow and is well tolerated because pressure is applied to the broad, well-muscled surface of the shoulder. Use of a single elastic bandage avoids uncomfortable pressure over the olecranon while again keeping the moment arms as long as possible. A turnbuckle splint may also be used to as part of the rehabilitation protocol (**Fig. 14**).

DISCUSSION

Results of previous outcome studies for total elbow arthroplasty (TEA) show promising results in specific patient populations, primarily the elderly.[20–22,29,30] However, limited activity restrictions, such as prohibition of lifting more than 5 kg and repetitive lifting greater than 1 kg, may not be attractive options to younger, higher-demand patients. Despite previous and recent studies demonstrating improved results,[6,15,31] the durability of TEA remains a concern. Multiple revisions progressively compromise remaining bone stock and sepsis may preclude reimplantation, leaving only resection or arthrodesis as 2 unsatisfactory alternatives.

Interposition arthroplasty is a reasonable and viable alternative for younger, more active patients. Long-term outcome series have shown that this procedure remains a practical option for this patient population. Cheng and Morrey demonstrated a 69% satisfactory result and 62% excellent or good result following interposition arthroplasty after a 63-month follow-up.[17] These results have been shown to be similar in both the posttraumatic and inflammatory elbow. The issue of instability has been addressed with the addition of distraction and external fixation, in conjunction with ligament reconstruction, and has yielded improved results.[16,17] Patients with advanced arthritis are able to buy time with interposition arthroplasty, and subsequent conversion to STEA in the future remains an option, although in the authors' experience, few patients request such conversion. Blaine and colleagues[32] demonstrated successful outcomes of TEA after interposition arthroplasty, suggesting that prior interposition arthroplasty does not compromise the results of TEA. While x rays of interposition arthroplasties may be alarming, radiographs do not correlate well with pain relief and functional outcomes, which are usually satisfactory and durable. However, surgeons and patients must understand that even an outstanding interposition arthroplasty will not equal the pain relief and motion of a successful STEA. Interposition is really about minimizing long-term, downside risk, at the expense of a shorter-term, excellent result.

Achieving good results depends on several factors, including

1. Proper indications: Elbow stability and preserved bony anatomy are absolute prerequisites for successful interposition arthroplasty.
2. Appropriate patient expectations: The surgeon should realistically discuss what can and cannot be achieved and emphasize that the goal is to achieve an imperfect outcome that affords adequate, although not total, pain relief and a functional, although incomplete, range of motion. Results have shown good pain relief and satisfactory range of motion, thus making it a good preprosthetic alternative.
3. Comprehensive joint release: An adequate capsular release must be performed.
4. Stable resurfacing of the joint surface: The graft material fixation should be firm and stable. It is not necessary to resurface both the humerus and ulna, and the radial head should be preserved. If not present, arthroplasty may be considered to improve elbow stability.
5. Careful wound management and drainage should be practiced to avoid complications.
6. If external fixation is used, the axis must be perfect. If this cannot be achieved with certainty, one should seriously consider removing the fixator. As mentioned, the authors no longer use a fixator for routine interposition arthroplasty and have found no difference in motion or pain relief.
7. Ligament reconstruction: Repair or reconstruction of the ligaments, using tendon grafts, if necessary, is absolutely mandatory. The goal of this operation is to create an anatomic

reconstruction with a new joint surface. Therefore, anatomic ligament and muscle reconstruction is mandatory.

Adherence to these principles can help to achieve a satisfactory and durable solution for the challenging problem of elbow arthritis while preserving future treatment and revision options, including conversion to a total elbow arthroplasty when predictable and successful long-term outcomes are demonstrated.

REFERENCES

1. Kauffman J, Chen A, Stuchin S, et al. Surgical management of the rheumatoid elbow. J Am Acad Orthop Surg 2003;11(2):100–8.
2. Morrey BF, Askew LJ, Chao EY. A biomechanical study of normal functional elbow motion. J Bone Joint Surg Am 1981;63(6):872–7.
3. Phillips N, Ali A, Stanley D. Treatment of primary degenerative arthritis of the elbow by ulnohumeral arthroplasty-a long term follow-up. J Bone Joint Surg Br 2003;85(3):347–50.
4. Gschwend N, Simmen B, Matejovsky Z. Late complications in elbow arthroplasty. J Shoulder Elbow Surg 1996;5(2):86–96.
5. Ingles A, Pellicci P. Total elbow replacement. J Bone Joint Surg Am 1980;62(8):1252–8.
6. Morrey BF. Complications of elbow replacement surgery. In: Morrey BF, Lampert R, editors. The elbow and its disorders. Philadelphia: WB Saunders; 2000. p. 667–77.
7. Volkov MV, Oganesian OV. Restoration of function in the knee and elbow with a hinge-distractor apparatus. J Bone Joint Surg Am 1975;57:591–600.
8. Verneuil A. De la creation d'une fausse articulation par section ou resection partielle de l'os maxillaire inferieur, comme moyen de remedier l'ankylose orale de fausse de la machoure inferieur. Arch Gen Med 1860;15:284.
9. Campbell WC. Mobilization of joints with bony ankylosis: an analysis of 110 cases. JAMA 1924;93:976.
10. Deland JT, Walker PS, Sledge CB, et al. Treatment of posttraumatic elbows with a new hinge distractor. Orthopedics 1983;6:732.
11. Ljung P, Jonsson K, Larsson K, et al. Interposition arthroplasty of the elbow with rheumatoid arthritis. J Shoulder Elbow Surg 1996;5:81–5.
12. Fernandez-Palazzi F, Rodriguez J, Oliver G. Elbow interposition arthroplasty in children and adolescents: long term follow-up. Int Orthop 2008;32:247–50.
13. Kita M. Arthroplasty of the elbow using J-K membrane. Acta Orthop Scand 1977;48:450–5.
14. Knight RA, Van Zandt IL. Arthroplasty of the elbow: an end result study. J Bone Joint Surg Am 1952; 34:610–8.
15. Nolla J, Ring D, Lozano-Calderon S, et al. Interposition arthroplasty of the elbow with hinged external fixation for post-traumatic arthritis. J Shoulder Elbow Surg 2008;17:459–64.
16. Fox JR, Varitimidis SE, Plakseychuk A, et al. The compass elbow hinge: indications and initial results. J Hand Surg Br 2000;25:568–72.
17. Cheng SL, Morrey BF. The treatment of the mobile, painful arthritic elbow by distraction interposition arthroplasty. J Bone Joint Surg Br 2000;82:233–8.
18. Manat P. Surgical treatment of the rheumatoid elbow. Joint Bone Spine 2001;68:198–210.
19. Wright P, Froimson AI, Morrey BF, et al. Interposition arthroplasty of the elbow. In: Morrey BF, Lampert R, editors. The elbow and its disorders. Philadelphia: WB Saunders; 2000. p. 718–30.
20. Cobb TK, Morrey BF. Total elbow arthroplasty as primary treatment for distal humerus fractures in elderly patients. J Bone Joint Surg Am 1997;79: 826–32.
21. Gill DRJ, Morrey BF. The Coonrad–Morrey total elbow arthroplasty in patients who have rheumatoid arthritis. J Bone Joint Surg Am 1998;80:1327–35.
22. Schneeberger AG, Adams R, Morrey BF. Semiconstrained total elbow replacement for the treatment of posttraumatic arthritis. J Bone Joint Surg Am 1997;79:1211–22.
23. Bottlang MR, O'Rourke MR, Madey SM, et al. Radiographic determinants of the elbow rotation axis: experimental identification and quantitative validation. J Orthop Res 2000;18:821–8.
24. von Knoch F, Marsh JL, Steyers C, et al. A new articulated external fixation technique for difficult elbow trauma. Iowa Orthop J 2001;21:13–9.
25. Jobe FW, Stark H, Lombardo SF. Reconstruction of the ulnar collateral ligament in athletes. J Bone Joint Surg Am 1986;68:1158–63.
26. O'Driscoll SW, Bell DF, Morrey BF. Posterolateral rotatory instability of the elbow. J Bone Joint Surg Am 1991;73:440–6.
27. Delamora SN, Hausman MR. Lateral ulnar collateral ligament reconstruction using the lateral triceps fascia. Orthopedics 2002;25:909–12.
28. Larson AN, Morrey BF. Interposition arthroplasty with an Achilles tendon allograft as a salvage procedure for the elbow. J Bone Joint Surg Am 2008;90:2714–23.
29. Lee DH. Posttraumatic elbow arthritis and arthroplasty. Orthop Clin North Am 1999;30:141–62.
30. Ramsey ML, Morrey BF. Instability of the elbow treated with semiconstrained total elbow arthroplasty. J Bone Joint Surg Am 1999;81:38–47.
31. Morrey BF, Bryan RS. Infection after total elbow arthroplasty. J Bone Joint Surg Am 1983;65:330–8.
32. Blaine TA, Adams R, Morrey BF. Total elbow arthroplasty after interposition arthroplasty for elbow arthritis. J Bone Joint Surg Am 2005;87:286–92.

Linked Total Elbow Arthroplasty

Donald H. Lee, MD

KEYWORDS

- Elbow • Arthroplasty • Replacement • Linked
- Semiconstrained

The choice between an unlinked (unconstrained) implant and a linked (semiconstrained) implant depends on joint stability and adequacy of bone stock. In general, in order for an unlinked implant to work properly, there must be adequate bone stock, intact or reparable collateral ligaments, and sufficient muscle strength about the elbow.[1] Linked implants can be used in elbows with intact bone stock and joint stability or those elbows with inadequate bone stock or joint instability. In the United States, linked elbow implants are more commonly used.

With linked implants, the linkage between the humeral and ulnar components allows for the transmission of joint reactive forces. Early fully constrained elbow implants have been abandoned because the significant joint reactive forces led to a high incidence of aseptic loosening.[2–4]

Linked elbow implants, compared with unlinked implants, provide improved joint stability and minimize stress at the bone cement-implant interfaces by allowing approximately 5° to 10° of angular (varus-valgus) and rotatory laxity at the ulnohumeral articulation.[1,5] These so-called sloppy hinge implants articulate or couple the humeral and ulnar components with some form of metal to polyethylene bushings or linkages. These modern semiconstrained linked implants have increased survival rates of elbow implants, but aseptic loosening secondary to polyethylene particulate wear, particularly in younger, higher-demand patients, remains a problem.[6,7] Elbow arthroplasty in these younger patients is not recommended.

Currently, the commercially available linked implants in the United States include the Coonrad-Morrey (Zimmer, Warsaw, IN, USA) (**Fig. 1**), Discovery Elbow (Biomet, Warsaw, IN, USA) (**Fig. 2**), Solar (Stryker, Kalamazoo, MI, USA) (**Fig. 3**), and Latitude (Tornier, Edina, MN, USA) (**Fig. 4**). The Latitude implant is a convertible implant that allows the implant to be placed as a distal humeral implant (hemiarthroplasty), unlinked implant, or linked total elbow implant.

Currently, there is insufficient evidence to identify the best type of elbow implant. The choice of implant is determined by surgeons' preference, their familiarity with the implant, and patients' particular circumstances.

INDICATIONS

The decision to perform a total elbow arthroplasty (TEA) should be made only after careful deliberation with patients. Patients must be willing to accept the lifelong restrictions associated with this implant. Patients are advised not to lift an object that weighs more than 4.5 kg and not to lift, on a repetitive basis, an object that weighs more than 1 kg[8] when using the involved arm after placement of a total elbow implant. This is a severe limitation on the operated arm but may represent a worthy compromise if the elbow is disabled by pain before the surgery.

Indications for elbow arthroplasty are similar to those for other joint replacements, including pain, limited motion, and joint instability, typically resulting from degenerative, posttraumatic, or

Funding for article: None.
Conflict of interest: Consultant, royalties (Biomet).
Vanderbilt Orthopaedic Institute, Vanderbilt Hand & Upper Extremity Center, Medical Center East, South Tower, Suite 3200, Nashville, TN 37232-8828, USA
E-mail address: donald.h.lee@Vanderbilt.edu

Hand Clin 27 (2011) 199–213
doi:10.1016/j.hcl.2011.01.004

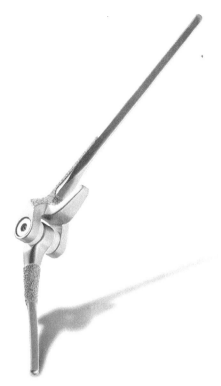

Fig. 1. Coonrad-Morrey total elbow system. (*Courtesy of* Zimmer, Warsaw, IN; with permission.)

inflammatory arthritic wear of the ulnohumeral and radiocapitellar joint surfaces. Elbow arthroplasty for an acute, severe intra-articular elbow fracture in elderly patients is increasingly used. A rare indication is conversion of an elbow arthrodesis to a TEA for functional improvement.

Rheumatoid Arthritis

In spite of the advances in the medical management of rheumatoid arthritis, the rheumatoid elbow is still a common indication for TEA (**Fig. 5**). One Swedish study, however, showed a decline in the overall incidence of upper limb rheumatoid surgery from 1998 to 2004 by approximately 30%. The most common areas for surgery were the hand (77%), followed by the shoulder (13%) and elbow (10%).[9]

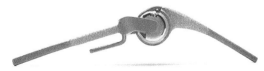

Fig. 2. Discovery elbow system. (*Courtesy of* Biomet, Warsaw, IN; with permission.)

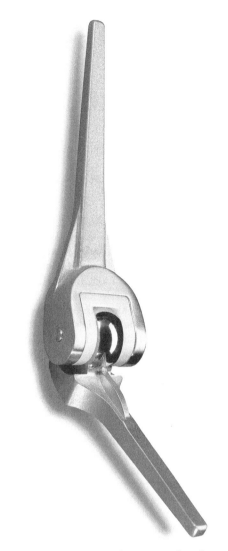

Fig. 3. Solar elbow system. (*Courtesy of* Stryker, Kalamazoo, MI; with permission.)

Osteoarthritis and Posttraumatic Arthritis

Osteoarthritis and posttraumatic arthritis are also common indications for TEA (**Fig. 6**). The results after TEA for osteoarthritis are typically less successful than those for rheumatoid arthritis, largely because of the younger patient population in this group, who place higher functional demands on their replaced elbow.[10] TEA in the setting of osteoarthritis is recommended for individuals older than 65 for whom other interventions have not succeeded and who are willing to accept low activity levels of the operated elbow.[10]

Acute Elbow Fractures

Anatomic reconstruction with open reduction and fixation of severe articular elbow fractures is

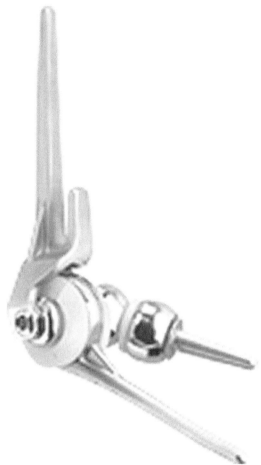

preferable, although not always possible (**Fig. 7**). In elderly patients with a severe intra-articular elbow fracture and in whom anatomic reconstruction is difficult or impossible, and likely to produce an unsuccessful result, primary TEA is an attractive option. Several studies have cited successful outcomes using TEA in this setting.[11–17]

Elbow Nonunions

Both intra-articular and extra-articular (supracondylar) distal humeral nonunions can be successfully addressed with TEA (**Fig. 8**).[18,19]

Other Indications

Other indications include patients with bone stock loss (after tumor resection, resection arthroplasty, or trauma), elbow ankylosis (posttrauma or postsurgical), and failed arthroplasty (**Fig. 9**).[20,21]

Contraindications

The absolute contraindication for a TEA is a joint with an active elbow infection. Other contraindications include an elbow with inadequate soft tissue coverage, one that lacks adequate muscle or motor power to flex (biceps function) the elbow, skeletally immature patients or young patients, or neuropathic (Charcot) elbow joint (**Fig. 10**). Relative contraindications include patients who are noncompliant or poorly motivated, patients requiring a fairly high functionally demanding elbow, or patients with a nonfunctional hand.

SURGICAL TECHNIQUE

Performing a TEA involves the following steps: (1) joint exposure, (2) ulnar nerve transposition, (3) distal humeral and proximal ulnar preparation, (4)

Fig. 4. Latitude total elbow prosthesis. (*Courtesy of Tornier, Edina, MN; with permission.*)

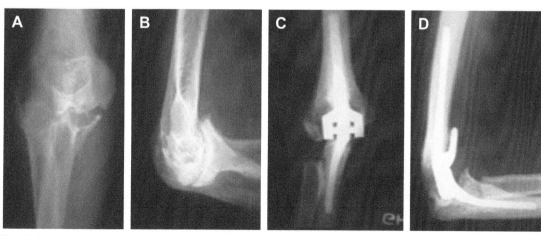

Fig. 5. Preoperative anteroposterior (*A*) and lateral (*B*) radiographs and postoperative anteroposterior (*C*) and lateral (*D*) radiographs of a patient with rheumatoid arthritis.

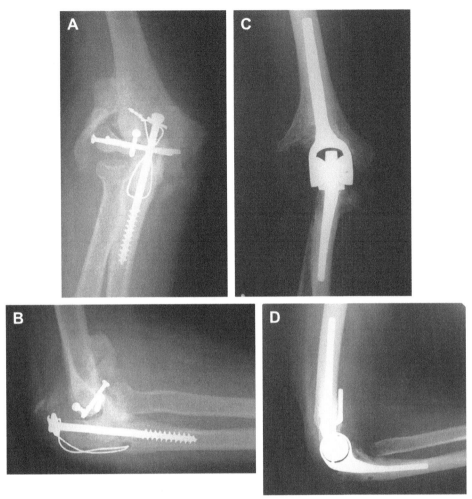

Fig. 6. Preoperative anteroposterior (*A*) and lateral (*B*) radiographs and postoperative anteroposterior (*C*) and lateral (*D*) radiographs of a patient with posttraumatic arthritis.

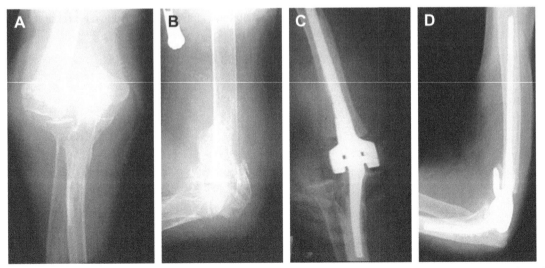

Fig. 7. Preoperative anteroposterior (*A*) and lateral (*B*) radiographs and postoperative anteroposterior (*C*) and lateral (*D*) radiographs of an elderly patient with complex intra-articular fracture treated acutely with a linked total elbow implant.

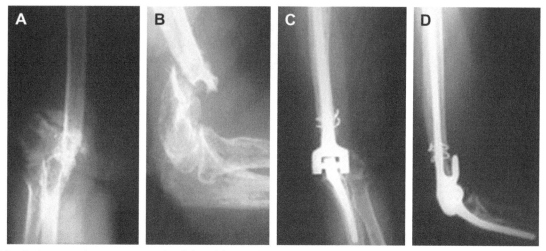

Fig. 8. Preoperative anteroposterior (*A*) and lateral (*B*) radiographs and postoperative anteroposterior (*C*) and lateral (*D*) radiographs of a patient with a distal humeral nonunion treated with a linked total elbow implant.

radial head preparation (if needed), (5) trial reduction of the implant, (6) assembly (if needed) and implanting the final components, (7) triceps reconstruction, and (8) wound closure.[22]

Several structures need to be addressed during the procedure, including the skin, ulnar nerve, triceps insertion, medial and lateral collateral ligaments, anterior and posterior joint capsules, and ulnohumeral and radiocapitellar joints. If a radial head replacement is performed, the posterior interosseous nerve needs to be protected.

General Considerations

Preoperative templating of the humeral, ulnar, and radial head (if needed) components is recommended. Templating allows a surgeon to review the preoperative radiographs, approximate the implant sizes needed, and determine whether or not standard or custom implants may be needed. Long-stemmed implants may be needed for revision cases or implants, with an extralong anterior flange may be needed for cases of distal humeral bone

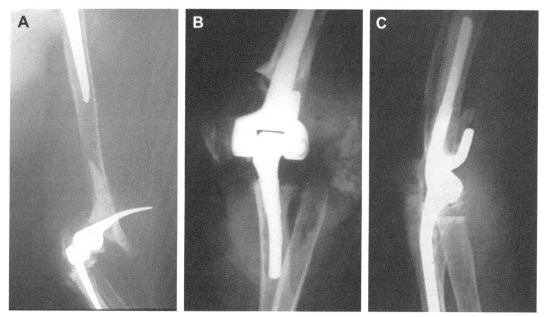

Fig. 9. Preoperative anteroposterior (*A*) radiograph and postoperative anteroposterior (*B*) and lateral (*C*) radiographs of a patient with a failed total elbow implant revised with a linked total elbow implant.

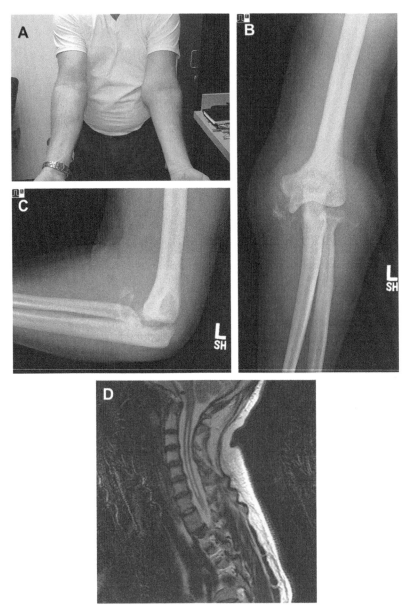

Fig. 10. Clinical picture of patient with a left-sided Charcot elbow (*A*). Anteroposterior (*B*) and lateral (*C*) elbow radiographs showing joint destruction. MRI of the cervical spine showing a syrinx within the spinal cord (*D*).

loss. The need for special equipment can also be determined at this time. The radiocapitellar joint is assessed to determine if the radial head is left intact, resected, or replaced.

Equipment Needed

In addition to the standard implant equipment provided by the manufacturer, extra instruments probably are needed for primary (**Box 1**) and revision cases (see **Box 1; Box 2**).

Patient Positioning

Patients may be positioned supine (author's preference) with the arm across the chest and a bolster for forearm support. A padded Mayo stand placed along the posterior aspect of the humerus can be used to support the arm during the surgical procedure. An alternative position is a lateral decubitus position with the arm draped over a padded arm positioner similar to that used for an elbow arthroscopy. A sterile tourniquet inflated to 250 mm Hg is used during the operative procedure.

Box 1
Equipment used for primary elbow arthroplasty

Sterile tourniquet

High-speed burr

Drills

Oscillating saw

Curettes

Pulse lavage

Appropriately sized humeral and ulnar canal cement restrictors

Pressurized cement gun with appropriately sized nozzle for the humeral and ulnar canal

Antibiotic impregnated cement (if used)

Fluoroscopy/intraoperative radiographs

SURGICAL APPROACH
Skin

In general, a posterior longitudinal incision is used. The incision is slightly curved around the tip of the olecranon process, either laterally (preferred by the author) or medially. Previous skin incisions should be used, if possible, to minimize the chance of skin slough and wound complications. If there is insufficient skin coverage, some form of soft tissue reconstruction should be performed at the time of the procedure or staged before the procedure.

Ulnar Nerve

Ulnar nerve complications are high. Although there may be some debate as to whether to not the ulnar nerve should visualized and transposed at the time

---

Box 2
Equipment used for revision elbow arthroplasty

Cement removal equipment

Flexible and curved osteotomes

Flexible reamers

Curved and straight gouges

Allograft bone graft

Instruments to obtain autologus bone grafts

Cerclage wire

Wires or Steinmann for antibiotic spacers

Screw extraction sets

Appropriate extraction tools for old implants

---

of surgery,[21] most surgeons recommend that the ulnar nerve be identified, mobilized, and transposed anteriorly at the time of surgery. In revision cases, it may be easier to identify the ulnar nerve proximally in an area with less soft tissue scarring and then the nerve is traced distally. Neurolysis of the ulnar nerve may also relieve any preoperative neurologic symptoms. In some revision cases, dissection of the humeral shaft may be needed. In these cases, the radial nerve should be identified and protected.

Triceps Insertion

Postoperative triceps weakness and insufficiency is common. If the triceps is reflected during the exposure, care should be taken to restore the triceps insertion. In some cases, such as distal humeral nonunions where the distal humerus is resected, acute distal humerus fractures, and revision arthroplasty, the triceps may be left intact and medial and lateral dissection of the triceps can be performed.

When a Bryan-Morrey approach is used, the triceps attachment and periosteum to the distal ulna are carefully reflected, releasing Sharpey fibers, from a medial to lateral direction, exposing the posterior elbow joint. One modification of this approach is elevating a small wafer of the posterior proximal olecranon, by using an oscillating saw, with the triceps. Alternatively, the triceps tendon and muscle can be split centrally, proximally, and longitudinally from its insertion onto the proximal ulna. The posterior joint capsule is usually reflected with the triceps.

Collateral Ligaments

The collateral ligaments can be left intact but are usually released from their epicondylar origin to increase joint exposure. If the collateral ligaments are to be repaired at a later point, they are tagged with nonabsorbable grasping sutures. Repair of the collateral ligaments and flexor and extensor muscle origins is somewhat debatable and is usually not performed.

Anterior and Posterior Joint Capsule

Joint capsular contractions can limit elbow joint motion. Both the anterior and posterior joint capsular contractures must be adequately released to restore elbow extension and flexion, respectively. If an elbow implant with an anterior humeral flange is used, the anterior capsule must be adequately elevated from its distal humeral insertion to allow the anterior flange of the implant to fully seat along the anterior distal humeral cortex.

Osseous Structures

The humeral and ulnar components must be placed at the proper depth into the humeral and ulnar canals, respectively, to replicate the normal elbow joint axis of rotation (**Fig. 11**). Placement of the components in a lengthened or proud position relative to the normal elbow axis of rotation leads to a flexion contracture and limits elbow extension. Conversely, placement of the components in a shortened position may lead to weakening of the elbow flexors and extensors, hyperextension of the elbow joint, and early loosening of the components.

Each implant system has its own cutting guides, reamers, broaches, and trial implants. Trial implants are used to insure that the humeral and ulnar components are properly seated and that full elbow motion is achieved before the final components are implanted. Meticulous preparation of the humeral and ulnar canals, the use of cement restrictors, and proper cementing technique are recommended. Readers should refer to the implant manufacturer's recommended surgical technique guides before using a particular implant.

Because of the inherent stability of a linked implant, the implant is somewhat more forgiving than an unlinked implant. Although placement of the hinged portion of the implant at the proper axis of rotation is important, the presence of the collateral ligaments or the humeral condyles is not as important for the linked implant as it is for the unlinked implant.

DISTAL HUMERAL AND PROXIMAL ULNAR PREPARATION
Humeral Preparation

After exposure of the elbow joint, sizing templates for the trochlea and capitellum are used if available. The center axis of rotation for flexion-extension is identified. Laterally this point is located in the center of the capitellum. When the capitellum is viewed from the lateral aspect of the elbow and imagined to be a circle, the center axis of rotation is located in the center of this circle (see **Fig. 11**). This point is the site of insertion of the

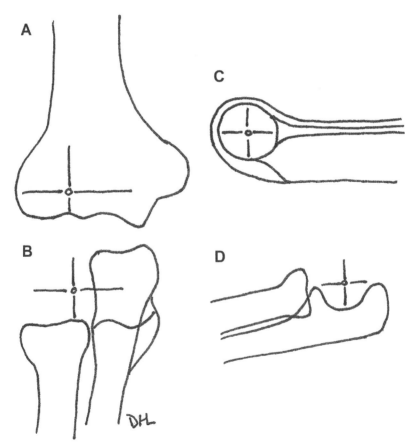

Fig. 11. Frontal (*A, B*) and lateral (*C, D*) projections of the distal humerus and proximal ulna, showing the location of the anatomic axis of rotation of the elbow joint. (*Courtesy of* Donald H. Lee, MD, Nashville, TN.)

lateral collateral ligament complex into the lateral epicondyle. Medially, the axis of rotation is located at the anteroinferior aspect of the medial epicondyle, also the site of insertion of the medial collateral ligament complex.

TEA Axis of Rotation

Some implant systems have humeral sizing guides, allowing the surgeon to approximate the size of the humeral component.

The humeral cutting guides for the distal humerus vary and can be an onlay cutting guide or an intramedullary cutting guide. With either technique, the initial cut usually removes a portion or a majority of the trochlea. The proper height (proximal-distal position) of the cutting guides is based on the axis of rotation. If an intramedullary cutting guide is used, a portion of the trochlea is removed, and the humeral medullary canal is opened, using a high-speed burr. That portion of the removed trochlea is saved for bone grafting posterior to the anterior humeral stem flange, if needed. The humeral canal is gradually enlarged by using serially sized humeral reamers. After placement of a properly sized intramedullary alignment rod, a humeral cutting block is attached to the intramedullary rod and used to remove the remaining portion of the trochlea.

Humeral reamers and broaches are used to further enlarge the humeral canal for the implant. Some implants have either barrel reamers or rasps to fine-tune the humeral cuts to further match the shape of the humeral implant. After preparation of the distal humerus, a trial implant is placed for adequate fit and placement at the proper height. At this point, the center of rotation of the humeral component should be aligned with the normal elbow axis of rotation.

Ulnar Preparation

Preparation of the proximal ulna is done with a freehand technique or with the use of alignment jigs that are placed parallel to the long axis of the ulna. These cutting guides are used to resect a portion of the greater sigmoid notch to match the contour of the ulnar component. Some resection guides that cut from a lateral to medial direction require the radial head to be resected before the resection of the greater sigmoid notch.

After resection of the greater sigmoid notch, the proximal ulnar intramedullary canal is then opened with a high-speed burr or a drill guide, then enlarged with a combination of the burr, ulnar rasps, and broaches to accommodate the stem of the ulnar component. The ulnar canal is serially reamed with reamers that increase in size. After

preparation of the proximal ulna, a trial ulnar implant is sized for fit.

Radial Head Preparation

Options for the radial head vary depending on the status of the proximal radioulnar joint, radiocapitellar joint, and type of elbow implant used. With degenerative changes involving the proximal radioulnar joint or radiocapitellar joint, the radial head is either excised or replaced. With unconstrained implants, the radial head is usually replaced. With semiconstrained implants, the radial head can be left alone, excised, or replaced.

An oscillating saw is used to resect the radial head at the level of the radial neck, after release of the annular ligament and protection of the posterior interosseous nerve. The forearm can be rotated so that different portions of the radial neck are exposed during the radial neck cut. The cut is performed perpendicular to the long axis of the radial neck. For implants that replace the radial head, the cut is made either freehand or with the use of a radial head-cutting guide.

Trial Reduction of the Implant

Trial implants are used to determine if the distal humeral and proximal ulnar cuts and preparation are adequate. The implants must be properly seated so that the hinge portion of the implant is at the true axis of rotation and that full motion, especially extension, is achieved. An elbow flexion contracture may be secondary to the components placed too proud or not fully seated or to an inadequate release of the anterior elbow capsule. If the components are fully and properly seated, further resection of the distal humerus may be needed to gain full elbow extension. Care should be taken to ensure that the anterior capsule is adequately released to allow components with an anterior humeral flange to fully seat along the anterior distal humeral cortex.

If the implant has an anterior humeral flange, the need for a bone graft beneath the flange is determined at this time, and the bone graft is prepared. The bone graft is contoured from a portion of the trochlea that had been previously resected. Roughening the anterior cortex of the humerus to help incorporation of the bone graft is another choice. Bone graft beneath the flange is not always needed. Care should be taken to ensure that complete seating of the humeral component is not impeded by a thick anterior humeral cortex or an overly large bone graft beneath the flange.

The final humeral and ulnar implants may have a plasma spray or precoating that may make the final implant slightly larger than the trial implant.

The surgeon may want to trial the final implants to ensure that these components fully seat before actually implanting the components with cement. Intraoperative radiographs or fluoroscopy should be used at this point to ensure that the components are adequately seated and placed within the humeral and ulnar canals.

Assembly of and Implanting the Final Components

The humeral and ulnar canals should be properly prepared before placement of methylmethacrylate. The canals are brushed, lavaged, and dried. Appropriately sized cement restrictors are placed in both the humeral and ulnar canals. The restrictors are placed approximately 2 stem diameters proximal to a fully seated humeral implant and distal to a fully seated ulnar implant. When cement restrictors are not available, morselized cancellous bone from the resected distal humerus or Gelfoam may be packed in the humeral and ulnar canals at the appropriate levels. The canal is dried and cement placed. The surgeon may choose to use antibiotic-laden cement. The cement should be placed in a fairly liquid state so that the implants can be placed within the canals easily. An appropriately sized humeral nozzle is needed for the cement gun to ensure that the nozzle fits within the humeral and ulnar canals. If the humeral nozzle is not available, a cut-to-size end of suction tubing, incorporated into the cement gun, can be used as a substitute nozzle.

If a semiconstrained implant is used, the humeral and ulnar components can be implanted separately and then articulated or implanted with both components preassembled. A radial head implant is usually implanted at the same time as the ulnar implant. A prepared wedge of bone graft, if needed, is placed posterior to the anterior humeral flange at this time. Care is taken to remove any excess cement. Final radiographs or fluoroscopy should be obtained.

Triceps Reconstruction

Triceps reconstruction is critical to maintain elbow extensor function. Techniques include a repair of the elevated proximal ulnar periosteum and triceps insertion with or without transosseous sutures into the proximal ulna. Care is taken to repair the ulnar periosteal sleeve with continuation of the repair proximally to repair the triceps fascia. The fascia is repaired as far proximally as possible. If transosseous ulnar sutures are used, a figure 8–type suture repair is incorporated into the repair. The ulnar nerve is formally transposed anteriorly at the time of triceps closure.

Collateral Ligament Repair

If a semiconstrained implant is used, the surgeon may choose to repair or not repair the collateral ligaments. Grasping-type nonabsorbable no. 2 sutures are placed in the lateral and medial collateral ligaments and common extensor and flexor origins. The sutures are placed through transosseous suture holes made in the lateral and medial epicondyles at the level of the central axis of rotation. In general, the collateral ligaments are not repaired with an unlinked implant.

Wound Closure and Postoperative Dressing

A suction drain may be used. The wound is closed in layers, and a bulky dressing is applied. Recommendations for immobilization vary from no immobilization to an elbow splint in full extension (to protect the triceps) to partial flexion. Active range of motion is begun within 3 to 5 days after surgery. The elbow is protected in an anterior long arm splint placing the elbow in extension or conversely a posterior long arm splint with the elbow in partial or 90° of flexion.

RESULTS

Early satisfaction and pain relief from semiconstrained TEA approaches 90% of patients in many series.[20,23] Improvements in design (semiconstrained design and anterior humeral flange) and cementation methods have resulted in fewer complications and better implant survival.[24–27]

Rheumatoid Arthritis

A 1998 10- to 15-year follow-up study of the Coonrad-Morrey TEA for patients with rheumatoid arthritis from the Mayo Clinic revealed a mean arc of flexion/extension of 28°/131° and pronation/supination of 68°/62° and 97% pain relief. The complication rate was 14%, and the overall survival of the prosthesis was 92%, with 86% satisfaction rate on the Mayo Elbow Performance Score.[26] In a 2000 study reporting on 51 elbows with a mean 4.2-year follow-up, patients with inflammatory arthropathy fared better postoperatively than those with fractures or posttraumatic arthritis.[28] A 1994 study noted a similar pattern of diminished performance of semiconstrained implants with implant survival rate for patients with inflammatory arthropathy was significantly better than for fractures or posttraumatic arthritis.[29] Overall, linked TEA results are good for rheumatoid arthritis, with high satisfaction rates for pain relief and function in the short and intermediate terms.[24,30,31]

Osteoarthritis and Posttraumatic Arthritis

A 1998 review of 5 patients with a 3-year follow-up of the Coonrad-Morrey prosthesis implanted for osteoarthritis revealed that 4 of 5 had complications, and revision was required in 2 of 5, although ultimately all patients experienced satisfactory outcomes.[32] High complication rates up to 43% using the Coonrad-Morrey prosthesis mainly for posttraumatic arthritis have been reported. The most common complication was early loosening.[8,33] In a review of 113 semiconstrained elbows, a lower rate of implant survival for implants was noted for posttraumatic conditions versus those for inflammatory arthritis. Specifically, the 3- and 5-year survival was 73% and 53% for the posttraumatic arthritis group versus 92% and 90% for the inflammatory group.[29]

Acute Elbow Fractures

A retrospective 1997 review of TEA as the primary treatment for distal humerus fractures in elderly patients revealed that 20 of 21 implants were intact at 3.3 years and the mean ulnohumeral arc of motion was 25° to 130°.[11] A 2005 review of similar indications revealed an average age of 69 years at the time of surgery, range of motion of 24° to 131°, and that 5 of 49 patients required revision.[13] Other reports show reasonably good outcomes after a TEA for acute elbow fractures.[12,16,17] A 2003 comparison of open reduction internal fixation (ORIF) versus TEA for the treatment of intra-articular fractures in women over age 65 revealed better outcomes in the TEA group.[14] A 2008 comparison study of primary TEA versus TEA after failed internal fixation or conservative treatment revealed no difference between the groups, indicating that TEA is feasible should ORIF not be successful.[15]

Elbow Nonunions

A report on 14 total elbow arthroplasties, both custom and noncustom, for distal humeral symptomatic nonunion showed a mean postoperative flexion arc of 100°, and 70% of patients reported excellent pain relief. Failure rate was approximately 30%, and 21% of patients had wound problems after surgery.[34]

In a 1995 retrospective review of 36 unstable distal humeral nonunions treated with TEA using the semiconstrained Coonrad-Morrey prosthesis, the mean patient age was 67.4 years (40 to 89). After an average 50.4-month follow-up (range 24–127 months), there were 86% satisfactory, 8% good, and 6% poor results. Average range of motion was 16° to 127°. There were 7 complications (deep infection, particulate synovitis, ulnar neuropathy, and polyethylene bushing failure), 5 of which required reoperation.[18]

A 1999 study of 19 unstable elbows treated with TEA for nonunion, severe erosive rheumatoid arthritis, traumatic distal humeral bone loss, and bone loss secondary to débridement for infection had an average follow-up of 72 months (range 25–128). Sixteen patients had minimal or no pain. The Mayo Elbow Performance Score average score improved from 44 preoperatively to 86 at final follow-up.[35]

A 2008 report of 92 elbows undergoing TEA as a salvage procedure for distal humeral nonunion found pain relief in 74% at a mean of 6.5 years postoperatively. There was a 35% incidence of reoperations, and 25% of patients required implant revision or removal. Factors associated with need for revision included patient age less than 65 years, 2 or more prior surgical procedures, and a history of infection. The rate of prosthetic survival without removal or revision for any reason was 96% at 2 years, 82% at 5 years, and 65% at both 10 and 15 years.[19]

Elbow Ankylosis

A review of 13 patients after TEA for ankylosis revealed a mean arc of 37° to 118° was ultimately achieved, although more than half the patients required reoperation, 3 developed a deep infection, and 3 required manipulation under anesthesia. In this group, heterotopic ossification prophylaxis was unsuccessful. Despite the high complication rate, the investigators concluded that TEA for anklyosis was an acceptable procedure in selected patients with reasonable expectations.[36]

In general, the improved performance of linked implants relates to the immediate stability afforded by the prosthesis with less reliance of surrounding soft tissue competence. Although this allows them to be used in a greater variety of indications, there is also more latitude for the surgeon to perform more aggressive soft tissue releases to enhance mobility. They allow more improvement in total motion compared with unlinked or resurfacing implants.[23,24,26,31] The stability assured from the hinge linkage allows for more aggressive capsular release, requires less maintenance of balanced tension in surrounding soft tissues, and may require less postoperative immobilization.

Complications

The complications of TEA include infection, prosthetic and periprosthetic fractures, aseptic loosening, bearing and prosthetic articulation problems, instability, nerve-related complications, triceps insufficiency, and heterotopic ossification.[37]

Infection

Infection after TEA and has been reported to occur in approximately 5% of cases (range 0% to 12%).[38] Infections can arise from direct inoculation of the joint, which can occur with ulceration of the thin posterior skin or hematogenous seeding of the joint. Patients with rheumatoid arthritis may be particularly susceptible due to history of corticosteroid or immune-modulating medication usage. In one series, 20% of patients with postoperative drainage ultimately developed an infection of the TEA. If postoperative drainage does not resolve within 5 days, the TEA should be débrided, cultured, and closed. Drainage appearing more than 10 days postoperatively is particularly ominous for infection.[39] The most frequently identified infecting organism is Staphylococcus aureus, followed by S epidermidis, although gram-negative organisms can also be identified.[40]

Prosthetic fractures and periprosthetic fractures

In a review of 27 fractured (17 ulnar and 10 humeral) total elbow components, all of the components fractured at a portion of the stem where the implant was unprotected by host bone. All humeral components fractured at the junction between the well-fixed proximal part of the stem and the less well supported distal stem, as did the ulnar components.[41]

The prevalence of periprosthetic fractures (humeral or ulnar bone fracture) is approximately 5%. In a review of 11 patients with a humeral fracture in association with a loose humeral component, treatment varied depending on the type of periprosthetic fracture noted.[42] Type 1 fractures occur distally around the columns or condyles, type 2 around the prosthetic stem, and type 3 proximal to the stem.

Intraoperative humeral fractures may occasionally be seen, usually of the condyles, and these may be treated with fixation at the time of index surgery. In one series, 3.8% (3/78) of total elbow replacements done for rheumatoid arthritis were associated with such fractures; one was excised, one treated with ORIF, and one was ignored.[26]

In a review of 22 elbows, the technique of proximal ulnar reconstruction with strut allografts for bone deficiencies, including periprosthetic fractures, is described.[43] Ulnar periprosthetic fractures were classified into type 1 fractures involving the olecranon process, type 2 fractures involving the area around the prosthetic stem, or type 3 fractures, which occur distal to the stem. Fractures distal to the stem in the setting of a stable ulnar component could be treated nonoperatively in some cases.

Twenty-five olecranon fractures and/or nonunions in TEA were reported.[44] The nonunion was treated by tension band fixation in 16 cases, excision in 4, and suture fixation in 2, and 3 patients with a stable fibrous union were left alone. Only 50% of the fractures that were repaired healed with osseous union, whereas 45% developed a stable fibrous union.

Aseptic loosening

Aseptic loosening of either the humeral or ulnar components must be distinguished from septic loosening. This distinction may be difficult, and laboratory studies of inflammatory markers, aspiration, or open biopsy should be considered before undertaking revision. Asymptomatic lucencies surrounding the prosthesis should be observed for progression and does not imply that the prosthesis is loose. A recent review of 125 Souter-Strathclyde (Stryker UK Limited, Newbury, UK) total elbow prostheses found minimal influence of prosthesis position on implant loosening, although by 5.5 years, 17% of prostheses had loosened radiographically.[45]

Semiconstrained devices have been reviewed with respect to loosening and have a surprisingly low rate of aseptic loosening. In a review of 78 TEAs performed for rheumatoid arthritis with 10- to 15-year follow-up, with radiographic loosening, defined as a progressive radiolucent line of more than 2 mm that was completely circumferential around the prosthesis, only 1 humeral component (1.3%) and 3 ulnar components (3.8%) were radiographically loose. Only 2 of these loose components required revision.[26]

Bearing and prosthetic articulation problems

Bushing and prosthetic articular wear is most commonly seen in TEA performed for osteoarthritis or fractures where higher demands are placed on the elbow. In a series of 41 TEAs for osteoarthritis, the polyethylene bushings wore out in 5% and were associated with particulate synovitis and osteolysis due to debris associated with the worn bushings. These cases were managed with synovectomy, débridement, and exchange of the bushings.[8]

In one series, 1.3% of Coonrad-Morrey total elbow prostheses required bushing exchange at an average of 8 years after implantation. These were mostly younger patients with an average age of 44 years at the time of the initial elbow arthroplasty. When the angle formed by the articulating portion of the ulnar component and the medial or lateral aspect of the humeral articular yoke exceeded 7°, bushing wear occurred. When the angle exceed 10°, patients may have been considered candidates for surgery, if they were symptomatic.[6]

One study reported on 10 patients with bushing and C-ring wear of the Coonrad-Morrey prosthesis requiring revision an average of 5 years after the initial procedure.[7] Particulate synovitis was found in all cases and revision arthroplasty was required in several cases, some requiring massive allograft. Complete dissociation of the components was also found in some cases due to the locking C-ring failure. The investigators recommended close follow-up (every 6 months) for patients who tended to place excessive demands on the TEA, typically for indications of posttraumatic arthritis or supracondylar nonunion. At the first sign of palpable synovitis, bushing wear, or osteolysis, a synovectomy and bushing exchange were recommended, because early operation was postulated to potentially obviate a more extensive later revision procedure.[46]

Instability

Instability of the semiconstrained devices has not been reported unless the linking mechanism disengages, such as in a snap-fit device, or as a result of the bushing and articulation wear (discussed previously), and in these cases revision of the components is typically required.

Nerve-related complications

The ulnar nerve is the most vulnerable during TEA; however, occasionally, posterior interosseous or radial nerve injuries have also been reported. Postoperative ulnar nerve involvement has been reported in 2% to 26% of patients.[47] Revision TEA poses particular risk to the ulnar nerve, which is often encased in scar tissue, and permanent ulnar nerve deficits have been reported.

Of some concern is a recent report of permanent radial nerve injury associated with ultrasonic cement removal from the humeral intramedullary canal.[48] A cadaver study demonstrated dangerously elevated temperature levels in the humerus, triceps, and radial nerve using an ultrasonic cement remover. Cold irrigation of the humeral canal was recommended intraoperatively, with consideration for exposure and protection of the radial nerve, if such a device is used.[48]

Triceps insufficiency

A review of 887 TEAs was performed to identify patients undergoing revision procedures for triceps insufficiency not due to infection; 16 of 887 cases were identified (1.8%).[49] The Bryan-Morrey approach had initially been used for 15 elbows and a triceps splitting approach in 1 case. Direct

repair was performed in 6 cases, an Achilles tendon allograft was used in 7 elbows, and anconeus rotational flaps used in 4. In 15 of 16 cases, the ability to extend against gravity was regained. The recommendation was made to repair the tendon if possible, use an anconeus flap if tendon repair was not possible, and use an Achilles tendon allograft for large defects, taking into account spontaneous resorption of the olecranon process.

Heterotopic ossification

Significant heterotopic ossification is uncommon after TEA.[37,47] In a review of 49 acute distal humeral fractures treated with the Coonrad-Morrey prosthesis, heterotopic ossification was found in 16% of the cases available for late review. Two of the cases had posterior bony impingement, which did not require revision.[13]

SUMMARY

With proper patient selection and advances in implant design, improvement in cementation techniques, meticulous surgical technique, and appropriate postoperative rehabilitation, linked elbow arthroplasty can provide high patient satisfaction and pain relief in approximately 90% of patients. Concerns remain about the use of this implant in young or high-demand patients.

REFERENCES

1. Gramstad GD, King GJ, O'Driscoll SW, et al. Elbow arthroplasty using a convertible implant. Tech Hand Up Extrem Surg 2005;9:153–63.
2. Ewald FC. Total elbow replacement. Orthop Clin North Am 1975;6:685–96.
3. Garrett JC, Ewald FC, Thomas WH, et al. Loosening associated with GSB hinge total elbow replacement in patients with rheumatoid arthritis. Clin Orthop Relat Res 1977;127:170–4.
4. Souter WA. Arthroplasty of the elbow: with particular reference to metallic hinge arthroplasty in rheumatoid patients. Orthop Clin North Am 1973;4:395–413.
5. Cooney WP, Morrey BF. Elbow arthroplasty: historical perspective and emerging concepts. In: Morrey BF, Sanchez-Sotelo J, editors. The elbow and its disorders. 4th edition. Philadelphia: Saunders Elsevier; 2009. p. 705–19. Chapter 51.
6. Lee BP, Adams RA, Morrey BF. Polyethylene wear after total elbow arthroplasty. J Bone Joint Surg Am 2005;87:1080–7.
7. Wright TW, Hastings H. Total elbow arthroplasty failure due to overuse, C-ring failure, and/or bushing wear. J Shoulder Elbow Surg 2005;14:65–72.
8. Schneeberger AG, Adams R, Morrey BF. Semiconstrained total elbow replacement for the treatment

of post-traumatic osteoarthrosis. J Bone Joint Surg Am 1997;79:1211–22.

9. Weiss RJ, Ehlin A, Montgomery SM, et al. Decrease of RA-related orthopedic surgery of the upper limbs between 1998 and 2004: data from 54,579 RA impatients. Rheumatology (Oxford) 2008;47:491–4.

10. Cheung EV, Adams R, Morrey BF. Total elbow arthroplasty in primary osteoarthritis of the elbow. J Am Acad Orthop Surg 2008;16:77–87.

11. Cobb TK, Morrey BF. Total elbow arthroplasty as primary treatment for distal humeral fractures in the elderly. J Bone Joint Surg Am 1997;79(6):826–32.

12. Garcia JA, Mykula R, Stanley D. Complex fractures of the distal humerus in the elderly. The role of total elbow replacement as primary treatment. J Bone Joint Surg Br 2002;84:812–6.

13. Kamineni S, Morrey BF. Distal humeral fractures treated with noncustom total elbow replacement. Surgical Technique. J Bone Joint Surg Am 2005; 87(Suppl 1):41–50.

14. Frankle MA, Herscovici D Jr, DiPasquale TG, et al. A comparison of open reduction internal fixation and primary total elbow arthroplasty in the treatment of intraarticular distal humerus fractures in women older than age 65. J Orthop Trauma 2003;17:473–80.

15. Prasad N, Dent C. Outcome of total elbow replacement for distal humeral fractures in the elderly: a comparison of primary surgery and surgery after failed internal fixation or conservative treatment. J Bone Joint Surg Br 2008;90:343–8.

16. Ray PS, Kakarlapudi K, Rajsekhar C, et al. Total elbow arthroplasty as primary treatment for distal humeral fractures in elderly patients. Injury 2000;31:687–92.

17. Gambirasio R, Riand N, Stern R, et al. Total elbow replacement for complex fractures of the distal humerus: an option for the elderly patient. J Bone Joint Surg Br 2001;83:974–8.

18. Morrey BF, Adams RA. Semiconstrained elbow replacement for distal humeral nonunion. J Bone Joint Surg Br 1995;77:67–72.

19. Cil A, Veillette CJ, Sanchez-Sotelo J, et al. Linked elbow replacement: a salvage procedure for distal humeral nonunion. J Bone Joint Surg Am 2008;90:1939–50.

20. Strauch RJ. Indications for total elbow arthroplasty. In: Lee DH, editor. Total elbow arthroplasty. Rosemont (IL): American Society for Surgery of the Hand; 2009. p. 23–31. Chapter 3.

21. Morrey BF. Linked elbow arthroplasty: rationale indications. In: Morrey BF, Sanchez-Sotelo J, editors. The elbow and its disorders. 4th edition. Philadelphia: Sanders Elsevier; 2009. p. 765–81.

22. Lee DH. Elbow arthroplasty: surgical techniques. In: Lee DH, editor. Total elbow arthroplasty. Rosemont (IL): American Society for Surgery of the Hand; 2009. p. 63–95. Chapter 7.

23. Watson JT. Outcomes of total elbow arthroplasty. In: Lee DH, editor. Total elbow arthroplasty. Rosemont

(IL): American Society for Surgery of the Hand; 2009. p. 109–41. Chapter 9.

24. Little CP, Graham AJ, Carr AJ. Total elbow arthroplasty: a systematic review of the literature in the English language until the end of 2003. J Bone Joint Surg Br 2005;87:437–44.

25. Little CP, Graham AJ, Karatzas G, et al. Outcomes of total elbow arthroplasty for rheumatoid arthritis: a comparative study of three implants. J Bone Joint Surg Am 2005;87:2439–48.

26. Gill DR, Morrey BF. The Coonrad Morrey total elbow arthroplasty in patients who have rheumatoid arthritis. A ten- to fifteen-year follow-up study. J Bone Joint Surg Am 1998;80:1327–35.

27. Morrey BF. Linked total elbow arthroplasty: the Coonrad-Morrey prostheses. In: Yamaguchi K, O'Driscoll SW, King GJW, et al, editors. Advanced reconstruction elbow and advanced reconstruction shoulder. Rosemont (IL): AAOS; 2007. p. 241–50.

28. Hildebrand KA, Patterson SD, Regan WD, et al. Functional outcome of semicon-strained total elbow arthroplasty. J Bone Joint Surg Am 2000;82: 1379–86.

29. Kraay MJ, Figgie MP, Inglis AE, et al. Primary semiconstrained total elbow arthroplasty. J Bone Joint Surg Br 1994;76(4):636–40.

30. Kelly EW, Coghlan J, Bell S. Five-to thirteen-year follow-up of the GSBIII total elbow arthroplasty. J Shoulder Elbow Surg 2004;13(4):434–40.

31. Morrey BF, Adams RA. Semiconstrained arthroplasty for the treatment of rheumatoid arthritis of the elbow. J Bone Joint Surg Am 1992;74:479–90.

32. Kozak TK, Adams RA, Morrey BF. Total elbow arthroplasty in primary osteoarthritis of the elbow. J Arthroplasty 1998;13:837–42.

33. Schneeberger AG, Meyer DC, Yian EH. Coonrad-Morrey total elbow replacement for primary and revision surgery: a 2- to 7.5-year follow-up study. J Shoulder Elbow Surg 2007;16:S47–54.

34. Figgie MP, Inglis AE, Mow CS, et al. Salvage of nonunion of supracondylar fracture of the humerus by total elbow arthroplasty. J Bone Joint Surg Am 1989;71:1058–65.

35. Ramsey ML, Adams RA, Morrey BF. Instability of the elbow treated with semiconstrained total elbow arthroplasty. J Bone Joint Surg Am 1999;81:38–47.

36. Peden JP, Morrey BF. Total elbow replacement for the management of the ankylosed or fused elbow. J Bone Joint Surg Br 2008;90:1198–204.

37. Strauch RJ. Complications of total elbow arthroplasty. In: Lee DH, editor. Total elbow arthroplasty. Rosemont (IL): American Society for Surgery of the Hand; 2009. p. 143–50. Chapter 10.

38. Gille J, Ince A, Gonzalez O, et al. Single-stage revision of peri-prosthetic infection following total elbow replacement. J Bone Joint Surg Br 2006;88(10): 1341–6.

39. Wolfe SW, Figgie MP, Inglis AE, et al. Management of infection about total elbow prostheses. J Bone Joint Surg Am 1990;72(2):198–212.

40. Yamaguchi K, Adams RA, Morrey BF. Infection after total elbow arthroplasty. J Bone Joint Surg Am 1998; 80(4):481–91.

41. Athwal GS, Morrey BF. Revision total elbow arthroplasty for prosthetic fractures. J Bone Joint Surg Am 2006;88(9):2017–26.

42. Sanchez-Sotelo J, O'Driscoll S, Morrey BF. Periprosthetic humeral fractures after total elbow arthroplasty: treatment with implant revision and strut allograft augmentation. J Bone Joint Surg Am 2002;84(9):1642–50.

43. Kamineni S, Morrey BF. Proximal ulnar reconstruction with strut allograft in revision total elbow arthroplasty. J Bone Joint Surg Am 2004;86(6):1223–9.

44. Marra G, Morrey BF, Gallay SH, et al. Fracture and nonunion of the olecranon in total elbow arthroplasty. J Shoulder Elbow Surg 2006;15(4):486–94.

45. van der Lugt JC, Geskus RB, Rozing PM. Limited influence of prosthetic position on aseptic loosening of elbow replacements: 125 elbows followed for an average period of 5.6 years. Acta Orthop 2005; 76(5):654–61.

46. Figgie MP, Su EP, Kahn B, et al. Locking mechanism failure in semiconstrained total elbow arthroplasty. J Shoulder Elbow Surg 2006;15(1):88–93.

47. Morrey BF, Voloshin I. Complications of elbow replacement arthroplasty. In: Morrey BF, Sanchez-Sotelo J, editors. The elbow and its disorders. 4th edition. Philadelphia: Sanders Elsevier; 2009. p. 849–61.

48. Goldberg SH, Cohen MS, Young M, et al. Thermal tissue damage caused by ultrasonic cement removal from the humerus. J Bone Joint Surg Am 2005;87(3):583–91.

49. Celli A, Arash A, Adams RA, et al. Triceps insufficiency following total elbow arthroplasty. J Bone Joint Surg Am 2005;87(9):1957–64.

Unlinked and Convertible Total Elbow Arthroplasty

Alexandre Leclerc, MD, FRCSC[a],
Graham J.W. King, MD, MSc, FRCSC[b],*

KEYWORDS

- Total elbow arthroplasty • Unlinked prostheses
- Convertible prostheses • Elbow arthroplasty

Total elbow arthroplasty (TEA) is still in its infancy if we compare it with other arthroplasties such as knee or hip. TEA designs have been evolving with experience; however, long-term outcome data remain limited. The designs of total elbow prostheses can be subdivided into 3 general categories: unlinked, linked, and convertible devices. This article focuses on unlinked and convertible prostheses.

PATIENT SELECTION

Rigorous patient selection plays a crucial role in the success of elbow arthroplasty. In the early experience with elbow arthroplasty, only low-demand patients with rheumatoid arthritis were considered to be candidates for surgery because of the high complication rates with the first linked designs. A better understanding of elbow kinematics led to improvements in prosthetic design and surgical technique. Improved outcomes in recent years has resulted in a broadening of the indications for TEA to younger patients with both traumatic and posttraumatic conditions.[1]

General Indications

As for all elbow arthroplasty designs, typical indications include rheumatoid arthritis or other types of inflammatory arthritis, idiopathic or posttraumatic osteoarthritis, osteonecrosis, hemophilic arthropathy, oncologic reconstruction, and comminuted distal humeral fractures.

Specific Prerequisites for Unlinked Design

Adequate bone stock and competent collateral ligaments are essential prerequisites for the use of unlinked total elbow arthroplasty. Functioning flexor and extensor muscle groups are also important; a good muscle balance helps to ensure the implant remains stable. In the absence of these prerequisites, the surgeon should choose a linked prosthesis.

Contraindications to Unlinked Arthroplasty

As in any joint replacement, active infection is an absolute contraindication to an elbow arthroplasty. History of previous infection, an inadequate soft tissue envelope, a nonfunctional hand, neuropathic arthropathy, and unwillingness of a patient to be compliant with postoperative and long-term restrictions are considered relative contraindications. Despite important advances in design, elbow arthroplasty should be used with caution in younger more active patients. Specifically for unlinked implants, inadequate bone stock and insufficient ligaments are contraindications; a linked device should then be used.

HISTORY OF ELBOW ARTHROPLASTY

Elbow arthroplasty was developed to provide pain relief, improve motion, and offer stability to painful, stiff, arthritic, and destroyed joints. The initial

a Division of Orthopaedic Surgery, Hand and Upper Limb Centre, St Joseph's Health Centre, 268 Grosvenor Street, London, ON N6A 4L6, Canada
b Division of Orthopaedic Surgery, Hand and Upper Limb Centre, University of Western Ontario, St Joseph's Health Care London, 268 Grosvenor Street, London, ON N6A 4L6, Canada
* Corresponding author.
E-mail address: gking@uwo.ca

Hand Clin 27 (2011) 215–227
doi:10.1016/j.hcl.2011.01.003
0749-0712/11/$ – see front matter © 2011 Elsevier Inc. All rights reserved.

implants were linked uniaxial hinges and although initially successful, were complicated by early loosening of the components. In 1977, Garrett and colleagues[2] reported a 50% rate of painful loosening with 3 to 5 years of follow-up. In 1981, Morrey and colleagues[3] reported similar results with radiolucent lines in 29 (40%) of 73 linked arthroplasties using the Mayo and Coonrad prostheses with an average follow-up of 43 months; 11 of these arthroplasties required revision because of painful aseptic loosening. With the advent of loose-hinge linked devices that allow some varus, valgus, and rotational motion, the outcomes of linked arthroplasties have improved; however, bearing wear and loosening continue to be a problem in younger more active patients.[4] With linked arthroplasty, forces and moments at the end point of laxity in the articulation create high stresses in the polyethylene of the linkage mechanism, which can cause premature bearing wear. These forces are transferred to the bone-cement and implant-cement interfaces, contributing to loosening.[5]

BIOMECHANICS OF UNLINKED DESIGN

Unlinked devices primarily rely on adequate capsule, ligaments, and tendons for stability; although the congruency of the implant surfaces also provides some intrinsic stability.[5] Unlinked implants allow soft tissues to absorb and dissipate some of the applied forces to the elbow. Load sharing between the implant and the soft tissues theoretically decreases the forces in the mechanical articulation and thereby lessens the torque at the cement-bone and cement-prosthesis interfaces.[5]

Several unlinked prostheses are currently commercially available and each has a different amount of intrinsic constraint by virtue of their articular shape (**Fig. 1**). A balance has to be found between less intrinsic implant constraint to reduce implant loading, and more intrinsic constraint to minimize maltracking and instability.[4] The soft tissue envelope has to be balanced and the components positioned properly for functional laxity of the joint to be within the range of structural laxity of the prosthesis. Normal kinematics have to be replicated to allow the collateral ligaments to remain taut throughout motion and for the muscles to provide compressive forces to enhance stability of the articulation. This soft tissue balance should reduce polyethylene wear, osteolysis, and thereby aseptic loosening.[6] Unlinked implants are now designed with stems to reduce the risk of loosening, which was common when the first stemless implants were introduced.

UNLINKED DESIGNS
Capitellocondylar

The capitellocondylar elbow arthroplasty was one of the first widely used unlinked designs and was first implanted in 1974.[5,7] It is no longer commercially available. Originally, the implant incorporated a radial head component but it was discontinued because of early concerns regarding radiolucent lines around the humeral component. These lines did not progress over a 2-year period and ultimately the use of a radial head component was not associated with a higher rate of loosening at long-term follow-up.[8]

From 1974 to 1977, the ulnar component was made of polyethylene, but it was subsequently modified to incorporate a chrome–cobalt stem with backing to prevent breakage of the ulnar stem.[7] The humeral component was also chrome–cobalt with an intramedullary stem that was designed to be cemented.[9] The long-term outcome of the capitellocondylar prosthesis has been excellent[10]; however, complications such as instability and transient ulnar-nerve palsies have been problematic.[5,11–15] Davis and colleagues[15] reported a 13% subluxation rate in 30 capitellocondylar arthroplasties. This high instability rate may, in part, be attributable to its design because the articular surface is shallow, resulting in less intrinsic constraint than a native elbow.[16]

Ewald and colleagues[17] published the results of 202 capitellocondylar implants at a mean follow-up of 69 months. Postoperatively, 87% of the patients were pain free. Flexion-extension and pronation-supination arcs improved by 24° and 35° respectively. The mean preoperative score of 26 improved to a mean postoperative score of 91 points. Ruth and Wilde[10] reported comparable results regarding pain relief, activities of daily living, and improved range of motion with 51 capitellocondylar elbow replacements at 6.5 years. The Kaplan-Meier cumulative survivorship analysis showed a 83% survival rate at 5.5 years with a complication rate of 45%. Ovesen and colleagues[18] reported similar results with 41 capitellocondylar replacements, reporting a survival rate of 83% at 6.9 years and a complication rate of 35%.

Pritchard ERS

The Pritchard ERS, which is no longer commercially available, had humeral, ulnar, and radial components. Van Riet and colleagues[19] reported that the most common cause for failure of this implant was incongruency of the ulnohumeral joint during the procedure. They observed poor postoperative radiographic alignment and incongruity in 52% of their patients (19/36), which was correlated with

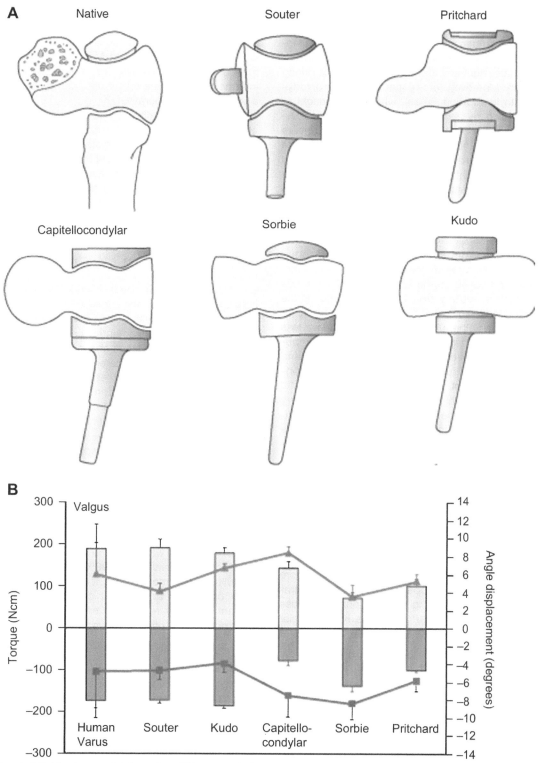

Fig. 1. (*A*) Ulnohumeral joint of 5 different unlinked TEA designs and their respective intrinsic constraint compared with the native elbow. (*B*) In an in vitro biomechanical study,[24] the kinematics of the human elbow were most closely approximated by the Souter and Kudo implants. (*From* King JGW. Unlinked total elbow arthroplasty. In: Morrey BF, Sanchez-Sotelo J, editors. The elbow and its disorders. 4th edition. Philadelphia: Saunders Elsevier; 2009. p. 740; with permission.)

early asymmetric polyethylene wear of the ulnar and radial head components. Radial head replacement did not compensate for misalignment of the ulno-humeral joint. This underlines the need to ensure adequate alignment and soft tissue balance during surgery. Moreover, some patients had ulnar or radial polyethylene dislodgement, which was thought to be caused by a poor locking mechanism.[19] The Kaplan Meier survivorship was 54% at 10 years (confidence interval: 40%–71%).[19] Inadequate implant design and nonoptimal surgical procedure both are thought to have contributed to high rates of instability, wear, and loosening.

Souter-Strathclyde

The Souter-Strathclyde implant (Stryker, Mahwah, NJ, USA) was developed in 1973 and first inserted in 1977. The vitallium-made humeral component is shaped based on the anatomic trochlea. It has a flat intramedullary stem that gains fixation in the supracondylar ridges.[20,21] It has a deeper trochlear groove than other unlinked designs that have less intrinsic constraint.[22] Long-stem humeral components are available for more complex cases and have improved survivorship relative to the short-stemmed implant.[23]

The all polyethylene ulnar component is very congruent with the trochlea and provides significant intrinsic constraint when loaded.[22,24] The implant can be converted to a snap-fit metal-backed ulnar component that changes this implant into a linked one, but this cannot be done without revising the stem unlike true convertible devices.[20]

Because of its geometry, this design has had less instability problems than other unlinked designs but loosening has been a more common problem. Landor and colleagues[25] reported the outcome of 58 arthroplasties with an average follow-up of 9.5 years. The Mayo elbow performance score improved from 30 preoperatively to 82 postoperatively. Aseptic loosening was the principal cause for the revision rate of 22%. The Kaplan Meier survival curves were 70% at 10 years and 53% at 16 years.

Kudo

The Kudo device has had more than 5 iterations since first designed. It is now marketed as the i.B.P. (Biomet, Warsaw, IN, USA). The type 1 and 2 designs were characterized by proximal subsidence of the stainless steel humeral component secondary to the absence of a sufficient stem.[26]

The type-3 prosthesis had a stainless steel humeral intramedullary stem added in 1980. Results were improved with a survival rate of 90% at 16 years.[27] Nevertheless, radiolucency around the humeral component at the intermediate (4 to 6 years) and late (11 to 16 years) follow-ups were common: 45% and 100% respectively. Clinical results were good with Mayo elbow performance scores of 81 and 77, respectively, for intermediate and late follow-ups, compared with a score of 43 preoperatively.[27]

The type 4 device had the humeral component changed to a titanium porous coated stem for uncemented use. High rates of stem fractures from fatigue, polyethylene wear, and metallosis contributed to poor performance of this design.[28]

The type 5 prosthesis has a humeral stem made of cobalt-chromium alloy with a titanium porous coating.[29] This design change reduced the incidence of radiolucency around the humeral stem[30] while still inserted using an uncemented technique. The ulnar component is either all polyethylene or has a metal backing with porous coating. Van der Heide and colleagues[31] and Tanaka and colleagues[32] reported the survivorship and clinical outcome are better with a cemented ulnar component than with an uncemented component. The humeral articular surface is shaped like a saddle, which permits medial and lateral translation of the ulnar component. The prosthesis requires excision of the radial head. The implant has good clinical results despite greater instability problems compared with other unlinked prostheses.[29,30,32–34] Recently, Thomas and colleagues[35] reported good results with 62 kind elbow replacements in 46 patients, at 8.5 years of follow-up. The average Mayo elbow score increased from 37 preoperatively to 86 postoperatively. The flexion-extension arc improved by 39°, from 60° preoperatively to 99° postoperatively, whereas pronation and supination respectively increased by 18° and 20°. The overall complication rate was 24%. The Kaplan Meier analysis showed a survival rate of 96% at 79 months and of 86% at 100 months with loosening occurring most commonly at the ulnar component. These implant longevity results are similar to what has been published in other previous reports.[31,32,34,36,37]

Sorbie-Questor

The Sorbie-Questor unlinked total elbow prosthesis (Wright Medical Technology, Arlington, TN, USA) (**Fig. 2**) is distinguished by the close match of its articular surface to the shape of the native joint.[38,39] The implant has cobalt-chrome humeral and metal-backed ulnar components. A humeral stem was added after early loosening problems of the original design, which did not have a stem. The radial head implant is a stemmed monoblock component. To date, there are no published data on the clinical outcome of this prosthesis.

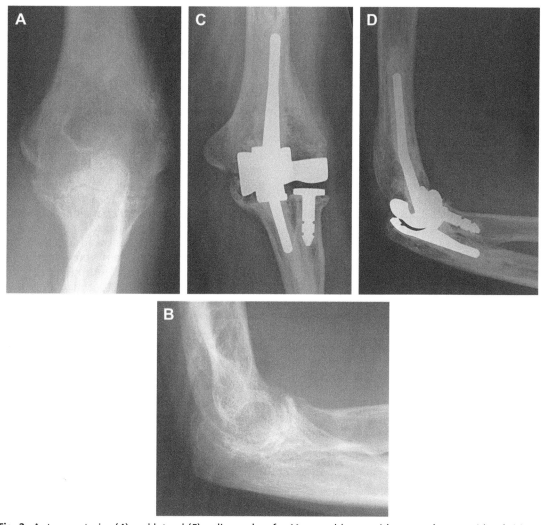

Fig. 2. Anteroposterior (*A*) and lateral (*B*) radiographs of a 41-year-old man with severe rheumatoid arthritis. At 10-year follow-up of a Sorbie-Questor TEA, anteroposterior (*C*) and lateral (*D*) radiographs show congruous articulation of the ulnohumeral and radiocapitellar joints with no sign of loosening.

THE ROLE OF RADIAL HEAD REPLACEMENT IN UNLINKED TEA

The importance of the radial head in TEA is still not fully understood. Retaining the native radial head or replacing it improves the stability in TEA. In a normal elbow with intact medial collateral ligament (MCL), the radial head is a secondary valgus stabilizer.[40,41] In the case of MCL insufficiency, the radial head becomes a significant valgus stabilizer. Many patients who undergo elbow arthroplasty have some element of ligament insufficiency. Rheumatoid arthritis causes the ligaments to be of poor quality and ligament damage is frequently present in posttraumatic conditions. Moreover, the collateral ligaments are often divided and repaired during surgery, which contributes to

their insufficiency. We also know that radial head resection can cause MCL attenuation and late valgus drift. Therefore, the radial head likely has an important role in early and late valgus stability in elbow arthroplasty. The advantage of radial head replacement has been proven biomechanically in an in vitro study for the Sorbie-Questor total elbow arthroplasty.[42] When a radial implant was used, the motion patterns of the Sorbie-Questor implant were similar to a native elbow. When a radial head replacement was performed, stability was further increased by simulated muscle loading, especially in extension where instability risks are the greatest. This phenomenon of dynamic stability was not observed when the radial head was not replaced. Clinical studies have also shown the importance of radial head replacement for other unlinked implants[8,43,44] and, therefore, its replacement may be an important factor for stability for this type of arthroplasty design.[8,42,45]

The radiocapitellar joint also has an important role in the transfer of forces across the elbow. It has been shown that when the normal elbow is in extension, 57% of the load passes through the radiocapitellar joint.[46] When the elbow is in pronation, the forces across the radiocapitellar joint are greater than in supination because the radius migrates proximally. Having the radiocapitellar joint to take a portion of the load distribution theoretically reduces the load on the ulno-humeral joint. The forces are dispersed across a larger polyethylene articulation, which lowers force transfer by the stems to the cement-bone and cement-prosthesis interfaces. In theory, this more anatomic spread of forces through both ulna and radius should improve the long-term implant survival with a decrease in wear, osteolysis, and aseptic loosening; however, this remains unproven.[1]

Restoration of an anatomic radiocapitellar joint is difficult. This is probably the reason why the early elbow arthroplasty designs did not include a radial head implant, or if they did, their outcome was suboptimal. Part of the difficulty is that proximal radial anatomy itself is complex. Radial head is inclined 15 degrees in relation to its neck and shaft.[47] Moreover, the radial head is not circular but elliptical and is offset from its axis.[48] Therefore, a round radial head implant with a straight stem cannot appropriately replicate normal anatomy.[19] A bipolar head can theoretically adapt to help accurately replicate the normal kinematics of the radiocapitellar joint and its relationship to the lesser sigmoid notch.[1]

Previously reported early total elbow arthroplasty failure in patients with an implant incorporating a radial head component may be caused by design issues and difficulties with precise implantation.[19] Advances in instruments and prosthesis designs may lead to improved outcomes of total elbow arthroplasty systems that incorporate a radial head component. Given the increased complexity of a 3-part verses a 2-part total elbow arthroplasty, further studies are needed to demonstrate whether the theoretical advantages of a radial head component are confirmed in clinical practice.

CONVERTIBLE TEA

A convertible total elbow device gives the surgeon the option to change from an unlinked to a linked articulation or vice versa without having to revise the prosthesis stems. Conversion can be done during the initial procedure or at a subsequent revision surgery. One system (Latitude System,

Tornier Inc, Stafford, TX, USA) also provides the option to convert from a distal humeral hemiarthroplasty to a TEA without removing the stem of the humeral component.

Rationale for Convertible TEA

Although a large proportion of patients who suffer from arthritis can be adequately treated with an unlinked elbow arthroplasty, other patients need a linked device owing to inadequate bone stock or collateral ligaments. Even if decision concerning the type of implant to use can often be taken before the procedure, it is advisable to have a linkable device available in the operating room whenever an unlinked total elbow arthroplasty is undertaken. Thus, if the unlinked implant is not stable or not articulating congruously intraoperatively, a linked design can be used instead. It is possible to change from an unlinked to a linked arthroplasty if the components have not been already cemented. However, repeat bony preparation will be required and is time consuming. In this particular situation, the convertible implant has an important advantage because it allows the surgeon to use a linkage mechanism that can be fixed to the same unlinked components for which the bony preparation has been done. If cementation of the stems has been performed and the prosthesis is recognized to be unstable, the convertible implant is even more advantageous because it is possible to quickly convert to a linked prosthesis without having to remove the stems. This versatility can also be very appealing in revision situations.

Another benefit for a surgeon and the team who work with a convertible device for most cases is the substantial experience they can acquire with one design; because they only have to get used to one implant, they will become very comfortable with it. For the hospital, it may also contribute to reduced inventories and cost, compared with having to deal with several designs.

Most patients who have an unlinked total elbow arthroplasty will have a good outcome. Nevertheless, some patients will develop elbow instability in the postoperative period, which can be a difficult problem to address.[49–51] When this issue presents acutely in the postoperative period, it can be treated by a closed reduction with a period of immobilization to allow healing of the ligaments. Afterward, the prosthesis may function normally; however, when instability is refractory to splinting, revision to a linked implant is the most reliable option because attempts at ligament reconstruction have not proved to be reliable. In this particular situation, a convertible implant can be linked with a minimally invasive approach while removing a well-cemented unlinked device and replacing it with a linked arthroplasty is very difficult with a high incidence of complications. This concept is also applicable to distal humerus hemiarthroplasties, which are increasingly being used for the management of complex articular fractures, nonunions and avascular necrosis. If, after a humeral hemiarthroplasty, a patient presents with instability, arthritis, persistent pain, or ulnar subsidence, there is a possibility to convert to either a linked or an unlinked TEA without having to remove the humeral component.

Convertible Implants

Two convertible elbow devices have been developed. The Acclaim (Depuy, Warsaw, IN, USA) is a cobalt-chromium implant consisting of a humeral component with fins and an ulnar component. The articulation is centered with respect to the long axis of the humeral component to compensate for the absence of a radial head implant. This creates lateralization of the ulna in relation to the humerus, leading to tightening of the medial collateral ligament. This is proposed to result in better balancing of the load across the implant to compensate for the lack of a radial head. The option to convert the unlinked joint to a linked one is done by partially removing the epicondyles and exchanging the bobbin to a polyethylene yoke. The polyethylene ulnar insert is replaced by a hinged component and a polyethylene pin mechanism is inserted. This implant system is no longer commercially available.

To date, very few studies are available on the outcome of the Acclaim device. Naqui and colleagues[52] reported good early results for osteoarthritis (average 57 months) on 11 patients older than 65 years. In this retrospective study, no instability or mechanical failures were reported and no implant revision was required. Bassi and colleagues[53] reviewed 36 cases, with most patients having rheumatoid arthritis. They reported no clinical or radiological loosening at a mean follow-up of 36 months. They had a 30.5% rate of intraoperative humeral condyle fracture, which did not seem to affect the final outcome. The humeral resection guide was redesigned to reduce the incidence of this problem.

The Latitude system is a cobalt-chrome modular implant that can be used as a humeral hemiarthroplasty or as a TEA in an unlinked or a linked mode (**Figs. 3** and **4**). The humeral component includes fins and an anterior flange that contribute to resist axial rotation as well as posterior displacement. A bipolar radial head articulation is optional. The cannulated axis bolt of the humeral component can be used to repair the collateral ligaments to the implant and adjacent bone. The metal-backed ulnar component has thick polyethylene and incorporates an extended coronoid process, which increases posterior stability. The conversion from an unlinked to a linked mode can be performed by adding a locking cap intraoperatively or during a subsequent surgery using a minimally invasive approach (**Fig. 5**).

SURGICAL TECHNIQUE CONVERTIBLE ARTHROPLASTY
Latitude System

The patient is placed in a supine position, with the arm across the chest. Prophylactic antibiotics are administered. A sterile tourniquet is used, which allows more proximal exposure if needed. A straight longitudinal incision is made just medial to the tip of the olecranon. Full-thickness flaps are developed as required on the deep fascia to preserve adequate cutaneous blood supply. The ulnar nerve is identified and mobilized to permit anterior transposition in a subcutaneous pouch. Excision of the medial intermuscular septum is important to avoid any subsequent tethering of the nerve.

Different deep approaches can be used. The triceps can be elevated from medial to lateral, as described by Bryan and Morrey,[54] or from lateral to medial as in the extended Kocher approach.[55–57] With either technique, continuity of the triceps with forearm fascia has to be maintained.[14,54,58] A triceps splitting approach elevating the triceps medially and laterally is another alternative. In certain situations, a triceps-on approach can be a good option and give sufficient exposure, especially when the joint is not too tight or when there is epicondylar bone loss. This approach, although not giving the same visualization as the other approaches, lowers the risk of triceps insufficiency in the postoperative period.[56,59]

The collateral ligaments are detached from the humeral epicondyles and tagged for later repair. Joint dislocation is now possible.

The sizing of the implant is a critical step. This is done by matching the anatomic spool size to the width of the distal humerus. Sizing is verified by ensuring that the native trochlear notch congruously articulates with the spool. The correct width will allow the radial head to align adequately with the capitellum of the spool when positioned in the trochlear groove. Four different prosthesis sizes are available for TEA, and 6 for distal humeral hemiarthroplasty.

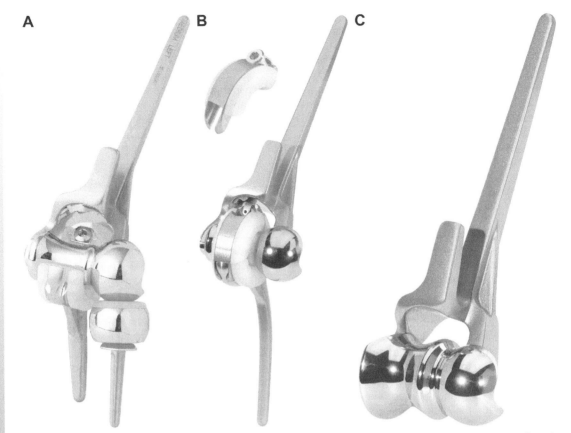

Fig. 3. Unlinked (*A*), and linked (*B*) and (*C*) hemiarthroplasty versions of the Latitude System. (*Courtesy of* Tornier Inc, Stafford, TX; with permission.)

An important technical aspect of the procedure is the replication of the anatomic flexion-extension axis, because all forthcoming surgical steps refer to it. Two landmarks are used for its determination. The center arc of the capitellum viewed from lateral represents the lateral point of isometry, whereas the anteroinferior portion of the medial epicondyle is the medial landmark.[60] A pin is placed in the flexion-extension axis. Removing the intercondylar portion of the distal humerus facilitates proper pin placement.

A burr is used to open the medullary canal of the humerus, and bone-cutting jigs, based on the flexion-extension axis, are used to accurately prepare the distal humerus to accept the implant. The humeral canal is prepared with rasps and flexible reamers if required. The humeral trial component can then be positioned.

Radial and ulnar preparation are done by using a cutting guide based on the anatomic spool and the ulnar diaphyseal axis. The anatomic spool is positioned in the trochlear groove and precisely aligned with the radial head. Adequate alignment of the radiocapitellar joint ensures correct rotation

for the proximal ulnar cut. Accuracy of the varus/valgus cut of the trochlear notch and the obliquity cut of the radial neck is established with the forearm axis guide.

The decision to retain or replace the radial head is made based on its condition and the ability to congruously align the radiocapitellar joint. When the radial head is replaced, proximal radius resection is made with a sagittal saw and a bell saw is used to cut the ulna from lateral to medial. If the native radial head is to be preserved, the ulnar cut is made from medial to lateral.

The ulnar canal is opened with a burr and intramedullary preparation is done with rasps and flexible reamers. A trial ulnar component is placed. After the radius has been broached, the correct-sized head is attached. The bipolar radial head can compensate and accommodate for 10 degrees of angular rotation but cannot compensate for gross malalignment of the radiocapitellar joint.

With the trial components in place, the stability and articular tracking of the elbow are examined throughout the arc of motion. If stability and

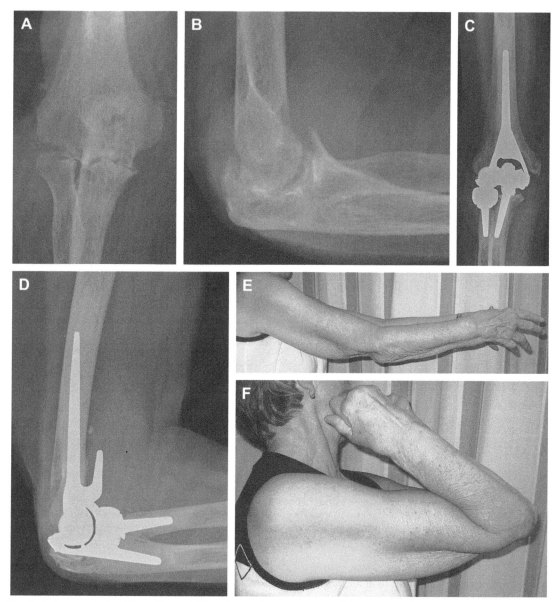

Fig. 4. Anteroposterior (*A*) and lateral (*B*) radiographs of a 44-year-old woman with rheumatoid arthritis. Anteroposterior (*C*) and lateral (*D*) radiographs 3 years following an unlinked Latitude TEA show congruous articulation of the implant. At 3-year follow-up, clinical pictures of the patient demonstrate good elbow extension (*E*) and flexion (*F*).

tracking are acceptable and there are adequate bony and soft tissue structures, an unlinked arthroplasty can be performed. If these prerequisites are not present, a linked articulation should be used. A close inspection of the radiocapitellar joint is necessary. If maltracking is occurring and it cannot be corrected by repositioning of the components, the radial head should not be replaced and one should consider linking the arthroplasty.

Cement restrictors are inserted and the medullary canal is irrigated with pulsatile lavage. Antibiotic cement is injected into the humerus, ulna, and radius with a cement gun. The definitive components are inserted. A cancellous bone graft is positioned underneath the anterior flange of the humeral component after the cement has hardened. The elbow is reexamined throughout its range of motion to evaluate for tracking and stability. If the implant is to be linked, the screw

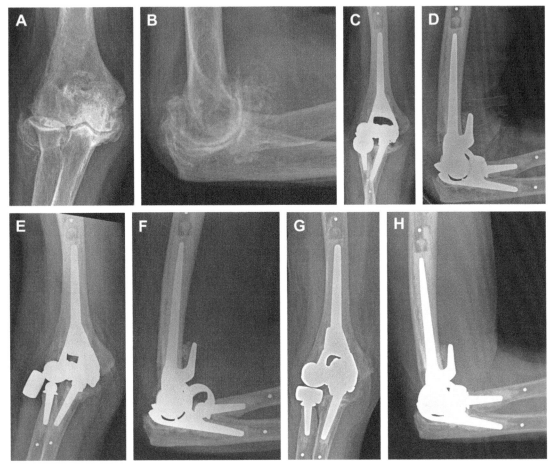

Fig. 5. Anteroposterior (*A*) and lateral (*B*) radiographs of a 59-year-old woman with rheumatoid arthritis. Anteroposterior (*C*) and lateral (*D*) radiographs 2 weeks following an unlinked Latitude TEA. At 6 months, anteroposterior (*E*) and lateral (*F*) radiographs show valgus laxity with radial head polyethylene dislodgment. Both medial and lateral collateral ligaments had failed to heal. The implant was revised successfully to a linked TEA without removing the stems. Anteroposterior (*G*) and lateral (*H*) radiographs show a stable linked Latitude TEA 1 year following revision.

in the ulnar component is removed and the ulnar cap is inserted and secured. Linkage of the implant is not performed until the cement has cured to avoid component displacement and suboptimal cement bonding.

The collateral ligaments are reattached to their anatomic origins using nonabsorbable sutures passed through the cannulated screw situated at the axis of rotation of the prosthesis. This avoids problems placing sutures in the weak bone of the epicondyles. These sutures are tied to the ligament on the opposite side of the elbow. The ends of the ligament sutures can be passed over the subcutaneous border of the proximal ulna to provide a temporary immediate artificial ligament in the early postoperative period, allowing time for the collateral ligaments to heal. The triceps is reattached to the olecranon if it was elevated.

The ulnar nerve is secured in the anteriorly transposed position. Drains can be used if needed. Finally, the elbow is placed in a well-padded splint in slight flexion.

Rehabilitation

The elbow is immobilized for 10 to 14 days to ensure stable wound healing. Active range of motion is commenced as soon as the wound permits it. Triceps precautions are required if the triceps was detached; only gravity-assisted extension should be allowed. A nighttime extension splint can be used to gain maximum elbow extension. Strengthening exercises are not started for a minimum of 12 weeks postoperatively, which ensures the ligaments had sufficient time to heal.

Complications

Complications of TEA include infection, ulnar neuropathy, periprosthetic fractures, triceps insufficiency, and soft tissue problems. Specifically for an unlinked prosthesis, instability is a concern, whereas for linked devices, polyethylene wear and stem loosening are the main issues in the longer term.

SUMMARY

Fully constrained linked total elbow systems historically had early loosening problems leading to poor long-term outcomes. Advances in implant design have improved the outcome of loose-hinge linked devices making them a reliable option for low-demand patients. Newer unlinked implants, designed to restore normal elbow kinematics, may lead to reduced polyethylene wear, osteolysis, and aseptic loosening. Newer unlinked devices may broaden TEA indications to include younger and more active individuals with adequate bone stock and competent ligaments. Instability remains the main concern with unlinked implants. Appropriate patient selection, improved implant designs, and more refined instrumentation may lead to a lower incidence of instability. Replicating the flexion-extension axis balances the dynamic and static soft tissue stabilizers, thereby enhancing elbow stability. Recreating an anatomic radiocapitellar articulation contributes to balance and spreads axial forces across the articulation, further stabilizing the elbow and potentially decreasing wear and aseptic loosening. Long-term follow-up results are encouraging even if they remain limited. Recently, convertible implants have added options by providing the best of unlinked and linked designs with a single device. Conversion between an unlinked and a linked arthroplasty can be performed either intraoperatively or postoperatively using a minimally invasive approach without requiring the difficult revision of well-fixed stems. Long-term outcomes are required for these newer implant designs.

REFERENCES

1. Gramstad GD, King GJ, O'Driscoll SW, et al. Elbow arthroplasty using a convertible implant. Tech Hand Up Extrem Surg 2005;9(3):153–63.
2. Garrett JC, Ewald FC, Thomas WH, et al. Loosening associated with G.S.B. hinge total elbow replacement in patients with rheumatoid arthritis. Clin Orthop Relat Res 1977;127:170–4.
3. Morrey BF, Bryan RS, Dobyns JH, et al. Total elbow arthroplasty. A five-year experience at the Mayo Clinic. J Bone Joint Surg Am 1981;63:1050–63.
4. Gregory JJ, Ennis O, Hay SM. Total elbow arthroplasty. Curr Orthop 2008;22:80–9.
5. Ewald FC, Scheinberg RD, Poss R, et al. Capitellocondylar total elbow arthroplasty. J Bone Joint Surg Am 1980;62A:1259–63.
6. O'Driscoll SW, An KN, Korinek S, et al. Kinematics of semi-constrained total elbow arthroplasty. J Bone Joint Surg Br 1992;74:297–9.
7. Kurtz Steven M. UHMWPE biomaterials handbook: ultra-high molecular weight polyethylene in total joint replacement and medical devices. 2nd edition. Burlington (MA): Academic Press; 2009. p. 143.
8. Trepman E, Vella IM, Ewald FC. Radial head replacement in capitellocondylar total elbow arthroplasty: 2- to 6-year follow-up evaluation in rheumatoid arthritis. J Arthroplasty 1991;6:67–77.
9. Rydholm U, Ljung P. Surface replacement of the rheumatoid elbow through a lateral approach. Tech Orthop 2003;18(3):258–66.
10. Ruth JT, Wilde AH. Capitellocondylar total elbow replacement, a long term follow-up study. J Bone Joint Surg Am 1992;74:95–100.
11. Ewald FC, Jacobs MA. Total elbow arthroplasty. Clin Orthop 1984;182:137–42.
12. Rosenberg GM. Turner RH nonconstrained total elbow arthroplasty. Clin Orthop 1984;187:154–62.
13. Trancik T, Wilde AH, Borden LS. Capitellocondylar total elbow arthroplasty. Two- to eight-year experience. Clin Orthop 1987;223:175–80.
14. Weiland AJ, Weiss APC, Wills RP, et al. Capitellocondylar total elbow replacement. A long-term follow-up study. J Bone Joint Surg Am 1989;71(2):217–22.
15. Davis RF, Weiland AJ, Hungerford DS, et al. Nonconstrained total elbow arthroplasty. Clin Orthop Relat Res 1982;171:156–60.
16. King GJ, Glauser SJ, Westreich A, et al. In vitro stability of an unconstrained total elbow prosthesis (influence of axial loading and joint flexion angle). J Arthroplasty 1993;8:291–8.
17. Ewald FC, Simmons ED Jr, Sullivan JA, et al. Capitellocondylar total elbow replacement in rheumatoid arthritis. Long-term results. J Bone Joint Surg Am 1993;4:498–507.
18. Ovesen J, Olsen BS, Johannsen HV, et al. Capitellocondylar total elbow replacement in late-stage rheumatoid arthritis. J Shoulder Elbow Surg 2005;14(4):414–20.
19. van Riet RP, Morrey BF, O'Driscoll SW. The Pritchard ERS total elbow prosthesis: lessons to be learned from failure. J Shoulder Elbow Surg 2009;18:791–5.
20. Dainton JN, Hutchins PM. A medium-term follow-up study of 44 Souter-Strathclyde elbow arthroplasties carried out for rheumatoid arthritis. J Shoulder Elbow Surg 2002;11:486–92.

21. Van der Lugt JCT, Geskus RB, Rozing PM. Primary Souter-Strathclyde total elbow prosthesis in rheumatoid arthritis. J Bone Joint Surg Am 2004;86-A: 465–73.

22. Schneeberger AG, King GJ, Song SW, et al. Kinematics and laxity of the Souter-Strathclyde total elbow prosthesis. J Shoulder Elbow Surg 2000;9:127–34.

23. Trail LA, Nutall D, Stanley JK. Comparison of survivorship between standard and long-stem Souter-Strathclyde total elbow arthroplasty. J Shoulder Elbow Surg 2002;11:373–6.

24. Kamineni S, O'Driscoll SW, Urban M, et al. Intrinsic constraint of unlinked total elbow replacements—the ulnotrochlear joint. J Bone Joint Surg Am 2005; 87(9):2019–27.

25. Landor I, Vavrik P, Jahoda D, et al. Total elbow replacement with the Souter-Strathclyde prosthesis in rheumatoid arthritis. Long-term follow-up. J Bone Joint Surg Br 2006;88(11):1460–3.

26. Kudo H, Iwano K. Total elbow arthroplasty with a non-constrained surface replacement prosthesis in patients who have rheumatoid arthritis. A long-term follow-up study. J Bone Joint Surg Am 1990;72:355–62.

27. Tanaka N, Kudo H, Iwano K, et al. Kudo total elbow arthroplasty in patients with rheumatoid arthritis. J Bone Joint Surg Am 2001;83:1506–13.

28. Kudo H, Iwano K, Nishino J. Cementless or hybrid total elbow arthroplasty with titanium-alloy implants. A study of interim clinical results and specific complications. J Arthroplasty 1994;9:269–78.

29. Kudo H, Iwano K, Nishino J. Total elbow arthroplasty with use of a nonconstrained humeral component inserted without cement in patients who have rheumatoid arthritis. J Bone Joint Surg Am 1999;81(9):1268–80.

30. Rauhaniemi J, Tiusanen H, Kyro A. Kudo total elbow arthroplasty in rheumatoid arthritis. Clinical and radiological results. J Hand Surg Br 2006;31(2):162–7.

31. Van Der Heide HJ, De Vos MJ, Brinkman JM, et al. Survivorship of the Kudo total elbow prosthesis comparative study of cemented and uncemented ulnar components: 89 cases followed for an average of 6 years. Acta Orthop 2007;78:258–62.

32. Tanaka N, Sakahashi H, Ishii S, et al. Comparison of two types of ulnar component in type-5 Kudo total elbow arthroplasty in patients with rheumatoid arthritis: a long-term follow-up. J Bone Joint Surg Br 2006;88(3):341–4.

33. Mori T, Kudo H, Iwano K, et al. Kudo type-5 total elbow arthroplasty in mutilating rheumatoid arthritis: a 5- to 11-year follow-up. J Bone Joint Surg Br 2006; 88(7):920–4.

34. Potter D, Claydon P, Stanley D. Total elbow replacement using the Kudo prosthesis. Clinical and radiological review with five to seven year follow up. J Bone Joint Surg Br 2003;85:354–7.

35. Thomas M, Adeeb M, Mersich I, et al. Kudo 5 total elbow replacement in patients with rheumatoid arthritis. A two centre 2 year to 11 year follow-up study. Shoulder Elbow 2009;1:43–50.

36. Little CP, Graham AJ, Karatzas G, et al. Outcomes of total elbow arthroplasty for rheumatoid arthritis: comparative study of three implants. J Bone Joint Surg Am 2005;87:2439–48.

37. Brinkman JM, De Vos MJ, Eygendaal D, et al. Failure mechanisms in uncemented Kudo type 5 elbow prosthesis in patients with rheumatoid arthritis: 7 of 49 ulnar components revised because of loosening after 2–10 years. Acta Orthop 2007;78:263–70.

38. Shiba R, Sorbie C, Siu DW, et al. Geometry of the humeroulnar joint. J Orthop Res 1988;6(6):897–906.

39. Sorbie C, Shiba R, Siu D, et al. The development of a surface arthroplasty for the elbow. Clin Orthop 1986;208:100–3.

40. Morrey BF, Tanaka S, An KN. Valgus stability of the elbow. A definition of primary and secondary constraints. Clin Orthop 1991;265:187–95.

41. King GJ, Zarzour ZD, Rath DA, et al. Metallic radial head arthroplasty improves valgus stability of the elbow. Clin Orthop Relat Res 1999;368:114–25.

42. Inagaki K, O'Driscoll SW, Neale PG, et al. Importance of a radial head component in Sorbie unlinked total elbow arthroplasty. Clin Orthop 2002;400:123–31.

43. Duranthon LD, Augereau B, Alnot JY, et al. GUEPAR total elbow prosthesis in rheumatoid arthritis. A multicentric retrospective study of 38 cases with an average 4-year follow-up. Rev Chir Orthop Reparatrice Appar Mot 2001;87:437–42.

44. Morrey BF, Adams RA. Semiconstrained arthroplasty for the treatment of rheumatoid arthritis of the elbow. J Bone Joint Surg Am 1992;74:479–90.

45. Ramsey M, Neale PG, Morrey BF, et al. Kinematics and functional characteristics of the Pritchard ERS unlinked total elbow arthroplasty. J Shoulder Elbow Surg 2003;12:385–90.

46. Halls AA, Travill A. Transmission of pressures across the elbow joint. Anat Rec 1964;150:243–7.

47. Morrey BF, Sanchez-Sotelo J. The elbow and its disorders. 4th edition. Philadelphia: Saunders, Elsevier; 2009. p. 11–38.

48. King GJ, Zarzour ZD, Patterson SD, et al. An anthropometric study of the radial head implications in the design of a prosthesis. J Arthroplasty 2001;16(1):112–6.

49. O'Driscoll SW, King GJ. Treatment of instability after total elbow arthroplasty. Orthop Clin North Am 2001; 32(4):679–95, ix.

50. Chiodo CP, Terry CL, Koris MJ. Reconstruction of the medial collateral ligament with flexor carpi radialis tendon graft for instability after capitellocondylar total elbow arthroplasty. J Shoulder Elbow Surg 1999;8(3):284–6.

51. Ring D, Kocher M, Koris M, et al. Revision of unstable capitellocondylar (unlinked) total elbow replacement. J Bone Joint Surg Am 2005;87(5): 1075–9.

52. Naqui SZ, Rajpura A, Nuttall D, et al. Early results of the Acclaim total elbow replacement in patients with primary osteoarthritis. J Bone Joint Surg Br 2010; 92(5):668–71.

53. Bassi RS, Simmons D, Ali F, et al. Early results of the Acclaim elbow replacement. J Bone Joint Surg Br 2007;89(4):486–9.

54. Bryan RS, Morrey BF. Extensive posterior exposure of the elbow. A triceps-sparing approach. Clin Orthop 1982;166:188–92.

55. Joshi RP, Yanni O, Gallannaugh SC. A modified posterior approach to the elbow for total elbow replacement. J Shoulder Elbow Surg 1999;8(6): 606–11.

56. Pierce TD, Herndon JH. The triceps preserving approach to total elbow arthroplasty. Clin Orthop 1998;354:144–52.

57. Wolfe SW, Ranawat CS. The osteo-anconeus flap. An approach for total elbow arthroplasty. J Bone Joint Surg Am 1990;72(5):684–8.

58. Morrey BF, Bryan RS. Complications of total elbow arthroplasty. Clin Orthop 1982;170:204–12.

59. Celli A, Arash A, Adams RA, et al. Triceps insufficiency following total elbow arthroplasty. J Bone Joint Surg Am 2005;87(9):1957–64.

60. Duck TR, Dunning CE, King GJ, et al. Variability and repeatability of the flexion axis at the ulnohumeral joint. J Orthop Res 2003;21:399–404.

Hemiarthroplasty of the Ulnohumeral and Radiocapitellar Joints

Scott P. Steinmann, MD

KEYWORDS

• Hemiarthroplasty • Humerus • Capitellum • Fracture

Most reports of hemiarthroplasty involve replacement of the distal portion of the humerus without replacement of the ulna. In 1947, Mellen and Phalen[1] first reported on an acrylic prosthesis that articulated with the greater sigmoid notch of the ulna. The design involved the humerus being placed down into the prosthesis and secured with wire sutures. The results provided patients with acceptable range of motion and excellent pain relief. There was, however, a less than 2-year follow-up period in their series.

In 1954, McAusland[2] reported on a series of 4 patients treated with a hemiarthroplasty. The prosthesis was shaped to duplicate the distal portion of the humerus and provided complete replacement for the epicondyles and the articular surface. It was also designed to be placed up into the humeral shaft for a press fit without additional cement fixation. The longest follow-up in this series was 3 years. All patients achieved excellent pain relief with no instability noted at the prosthesis-ulnar articulation.

In 1965, Barr and Eaton[3] presented a case report of a 30-year-old auto mechanic who had a previous nonunion of the distal humeral fracture with malalignment of the articular surfaces. The patient had resection of the comminuted distal humeral nonunion and replacement with a custom-made Vitallium prosthesis. The prosthesis itself was a press fit design that was modeled after an early hip nail and was seated with a mallet. Screw fixation was done through the shaft of the humerus and the prosthesis similar to locking screws in a femoral nail. The patient was followed up for 4 years and returned to an active manual labor career, putting severe stress on the prosthesis. At 4-year follow-up, one of the screws had broken but his elbow was symptom free.

Shrifin and Johnson[4] presented a 20-year follow-up of a patient who had undergone an elbow hemiarthroplasty in 1965 in a case report. They treated a 19-year-old man who had a comminuted distal humeral fracture treated by open reduction internal fixation complicated by subsequent infection. Later that year after the fracture had been treated, the nonunion of the distal humeral fracture was resected and a custom Vitallium endoprosthesis was implanted. At final follow-up at 20 years, the patient was satisfied and had returned to full activity.

Following these encouraging series of case reports, the largest series in the literature on hemiarthroplasty of the elbow was published by Street and Stevens[5] in 1974. They reported on 10 patients who had undergone an endoprosthetic replacement of the distal part of the humerus, including 5 with posttraumatic lesions, 3 with rheumatoid arthritis, and 2 with ankylosis secondary to hemophilia. The prosthesis was made of stainless steel or titanium and was essentially a cap resurfacing of the distal humerus. This U-shaped prosthesis was placed into the elbow from a medial approach with takedown of the medial collateral ligament while preserving the lateral collateral ligament. The distal articular surface was removed with a hand-held burr, and the prosthesis itself was driven with a mallet across the distal articular surface of the humerus in a press fit manner. No cement, pins, or screws were used to maintain the position of

Department of Orthopedic Surgery, Mayo Clinic, 200 1st Street SW, Rochester, MN 55905, USA
E-mail address: steinmann.scott@mayo.edu

Hand Clin 27 (2011) 229–232
doi:10.1016/j.hcl.2011.01.006
0749-0712/11/$ – see front matter © 2011 Elsevier Inc. All rights reserved.

the prosthesis. Because of its resurfacing nature, the attachment site of the medial collateral ligament was preserved and was reconstructed at the end of the procedure.

In their report, the investigators presented a 7-year follow-up in 1 patient who was an electrician who had returned to full work activity and reported no pain or disability. Loosening of the prosthesis or instability of the elbow joint did not occur in any of the 10 patients. The investigators concluded that hemiarthroplasty of the elbow seems to offer satisfactory pain relief.

After the report by Street and Stevens[5] on the results of hemiarthroplasty for the elbow, little was written on the subject of hemiarthroplasty until the 1990s. It would seem that enthusiasm for the procedure had waned. During the same period, the initial total elbow arthroplasty designs had been developed and many reports had described the techniques and successful results of total elbow arthroplasty.

It was not until 1999 that the next report on the use of hemiarthroplasty for the elbow was published. Swoboda and Scott[6] reported on the use of the Ewald capitellocondylar prosthesis in hemiarthroplasty. As compared with Ewald's report on total elbow arthroplasty, in which the average range of motion was from 37° to 118°, in this small group of 7 patients treated by Swoboda and Scott, the postoperative range of motion was only 60° to 98°. The investigators questioned whether ulnar erosion might progress long-term in patients with rheumatoid arthritis and whether these patients might ultimately require implantation of an ulnar component.

Elbow hemiarthroplasty has been used as a treatment of distal humeral fracture in the elderly patient. Adolfsson and Hammer[7] reported on a small series of 4 women, with an average age of 80 years, who had suffered a distal humeral intra-articular fracture. In their series, the Kudo humeral component was used. At a short follow-up of 10 months, all 4 patients had significant pain relief and had been using the extremity for daily activities. No instability of the ulnohumeral joint or implant loosening was reported.

In 2005, Parsons and colleagues[8] reported short-term data on 8 patients who underwent hemiarthroplasty with the Sorbie prosthesis (Wright Medical Technology, Inc, Arlington, TN, USA) (**Fig. 1**). Of these patients, 4 were treated for an acute fracture and 4 for nonacute trauma involving failure of fixation or nonunion. All patients had significantly less pain postoperatively; notably, the patients in the acute trauma group had less pain than the nonacute patients. Although the follow-up was relatively short, no patient in this

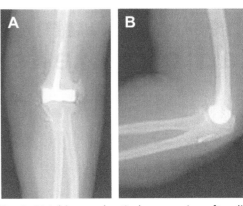

Fig. 1. Distal humeral articular nonunion after distal humeral hemiarthroplasty with the Sorbie implant. Successful 1-year outcome (*A, B*). (*From* Throckmorton TW, Zarkadas PC, Steinmann SP. Distal humeral fractures [review]. Hand Clin 2007;23(4):466, vi; with permission.)

series developed sepsis, loosening, or instability of the prosthesis.

INDICATIONS AND OUTCOMES FOR HEMIARTHROPLASTY OF THE ULNOHUMERAL JOINT

There are little data in the literature to guide the elbow surgeon in the proper indications and contraindications of hemiarthroplasty. Although little has been written on the subject, a common theme is that pain relief is significant, with rare loosening or instability of the implant.

An ideal indication for hemiarthroplasty of the elbow is the patient with rheumatoid arthritis who chooses to remain active. Such patients who have preservation of their humeral and ulnar bone stock with loss of only the cartilaginous joint space may be potential candidates for resurfacing of the distal humerus.

A second group of patients who might benefit from hemiarthroplasty are those with a low condylar shear fracture of the articular surface. In the case of low distal humeral fractures, the medial and lateral columns are often preserved, or if fractured, reconstruction of the columns can be achieved.

The third group of patients who can be considered for hemiarthroplasty are those who have failed open reduction internal fixation or nonunion of a low distal humeral fracture.

A relative contraindication for distal humeral replacement might be in the very elderly patient population. These patients have been shown to do relatively well after total elbow arthroplasty, which is a more straightforward procedure and is technically easier to perform.

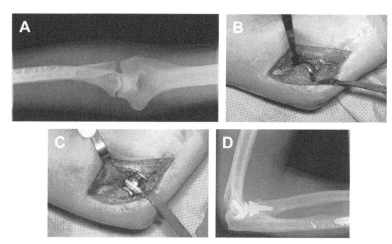

Fig. 2. (*A*) Anteroposterior radiograph of elbow after resection of the radial head for Essex-Lopresti injury in a 50-year-old man. (*B*) The elbow during surgery after replacement of the capitellum and (*C*) after replacement of the capitellum and radial head. (*D*) Postoperative lateral radiograph after radiocapitellar replacement.

The author has used distal humeral hemiarthroplasty for a mixed population of patients, including patients with nonunion, posttraumatic arthritis, chronic fracture-dislocation, and rheumatoid arthritis. In a recent review at the author's institution, the overall Mayo Elbow Performance score was 74.5 points after hemiarthroplasty of the elbow, correlating with a fair outcome. Most patients gained a functional range of motion. A revision rate of 16.7% was noted, but most patients had multiple prior surgeries for trauma, which may have put them at a higher risk for complications.

RADIOCAPITELLAR ARTHROPLASTY

Another hemiarthroplasty involves replacement of the radiocapitellar joint. This joint is a relatively small area of study, but recent advancements in technology have allowed for arthroplastyin this region. In cases of capitellar cartilage damage associated with radial head fracture or radiocapitellar arthrosis, the capitellum can be replaced along with the radial head (**Fig. 2**). Only a few designs are available to orthopedic surgeons, with limited follow-up. Heijink and colleagues[9] reported on the use of such a device in 3 patients. At several years' follow-up, the replacements had functioned effectively with no dissociation or loosening.

Unlike radial head replacement, which can be performed routinely without detachment of the lateral ligamentous structures, capitellar replacement in some patients requires detachment and repair of the lateral ligamentous structures. This requirement makes the procedure morecomplicated and introduces the possibility of postoperative elbow instability. In the author's experience, neither capitellar component loosening nor elbow instability has been found to occur in follow-up if attention is paid to lateral ligament integrity at the end of the procedure. The capitellar implant may be subjected to more compressive forces than shear forces, similar to the glenosphere in reverse total shoulder arthroplasty. Just as primarily compressive forces on the glenosphere have resulted in low loosening rates in reverse total shoulder arthroplasty, perhaps similar low loosening rates will be found to occur in association with capitellar implants after longer follow-up.

Radiocapitellar replacement remains a new technology, with only short-term scientific investigation reported in the literature. Further follow-up with long-term observation will be needed before making a general recommendation for its use.

REFERENCES

1. Mellen RH, Phalen GS. Arthroplasty of the elbow by replacement of the distal portion of the humerus with an acrylic prosthesis. J Bone Joint Surg Am 1947;29:348–53.
2. McAusland WR. Replacement of the lower end of the humerus with a prosthesis: a report of four cases. West J Surg Obstet Gynecol 1954;62(11):557–66.
3. Barr JS, Eaton RG. Elbow reconstruction with a new prosthesis to replace the distal end of the humerus. A case report. J Bone Joint Surg Am 1965;47(7):1408–13.
4. Shrifin PG, Johnson DP. Elbow hemiarthroplasty with 20-year follow-up study. A case report and literature review. Clin Orthop 1990;254:128–33.
5. Street DM, Stevens PS. A humeral replacement prosthesis for the elbow: results in ten elbows. J Bone Joint Surg Am 1974;56(6):1147–58.

6. Swoboda B, Scott RD. Humeral hemiarthroplasty of the elbow joint in young patients with rheumatoid arthritis. A report on 7 arthroplasties. J Arthroplasty 1999;14(5):553–9.

7. Adolfsson L, Hammer R. Elbow hemiarthroplasty for acute reconstruction of intraarticular distal humerus fractures. A preliminary report involving 4 patients. Acta Orthop 2006;77(5):785–7.

8. Parsons M, O'Brien RJ, Hughes JS. Elbow hemiarthroplasty for acute and salvage reconstruction of intra-articular distal humerus fractures. Tech Shoulder Elbow Surg 2005;6(2):87–97.

9. Heijink A, Morrey BF, Cooney WP. Radiocapitellar hemiarthroplasty for radiocapitellar arthritis: a report of three cases. J Shoulder Elbow Surg 2008;17(2): e12–5.

Index

Note: Page numbers of article titles are in **boldface** type.

A

Ankylosis, linked total elbow arthroplasty in, 209
Arthritis, of elbow, arthroscopy for, **171–178**
    diagnostic imaging in, 171–172
    historical perspective on, 187–188
    history and physical examination in, 171
    osteocapsular debridement for, **165–170**
    surgery in, 172
        anterior portals for, 173–175
        anterior procedures in, 173, 174, 175
        arthroscopic technique in, 172–173
        posterior portal placement for, 175–176,
          177
        postoperative rehabilitation following,
          176–177
   posttraumatic, and primary osteoarthritis, of
      elbow, **131–137**
   linkedtotal elbow arthroplasty in, 209
   rheumatoid. See *Rheumatoid arthritis*.
Arthrodesis, of elbow, **179–186**
    authors' experience with, 181–183
    case example of, 183–184, 185
    discussion of, 184–186
    indications for, 179
    literature review of, 179–181
    principles of, contribution by authors to, 180
    surgical technique for, authors' experience
      with, 181
        important observations regarding, 180
        positioning for, 181–182
        postoperative outcomes of, 183
Arthropathy, hemophilic, of elbow, **151–163**
Arthroplasty, distraction interposition, in rheumatoid
    arthritis, 144–145
   interposition, of elbow, **187–197**
   linked. See *Total elbow arthroplasty, linked*.
   of elbow, history of, 215–216
   radial head, 135
   total elbow. See *Total elbow arthroplasty*.
   unlinked. See *Total elbow arthroplasty, unlinked*.
Arthroscopy, for arthritis of elbow, **171–178**

C

Capitellocondylar unlinked total elbow arthroplasty,
   216
Convertible total elbow arthroplasty. See *Total elbow
   arthroplasty, convertible*.
Cubital tunnel syndrome, 165

D

Distraction interposition arthroplasty, in rheumatoid
   arthritis, 144–145

E

Elbow, acute fractures of, linked total elbow implant
   in, 200–201, 202
   arthritis of, arthroscopy for, **171–178**
      osteocapsular debridement for, **165–170**
   arthrodesis of, **179–186**
   arthroplasty of, history of, 215–216
   axis rotation of, axis pin through, 191, 193
   fractures of. See *Fractures*.
   interposition arthroplasty of, **187–197**
   nonunion of, total elbow arthroplasty in, 201, 203
   primary osteoarthritis and posttraumatic arthritis
     of, **131–137**
   rheumatoid arthritis of, **139–150**
Elbow system, Coonrad-Morrey, 199, 200
   discovery, 199, 200
   solar, 199, 200

F

Fractures, acute, linked total elbow arthroplasty in,
   209
      linked total elbow implant in, 200–201, 202
   periprosthetic, following linked total elbow
     arthroplasty, 210
   prosthetic, following linked total elbow
     arthroplasty, 210

H

Hemiarthroplasty, of ulnohumeral and radiocapitellar
   joints, **229–232**
     case reports of, 229–230
Hemophilic arthropathy, of elbow, **151–163**
   causes of, 152
   chronic stage of, 151
   clinical features of, 152–154
   clinical management of, 155–157
   joint replacement arthroplasty in, 159–160
   management options for, 157–158
   multidisciplinary approach to, 160–162
   pathophysiology of, 151–152
   preoperative and perioperative considerations
     in, 160

Hand Clin 27 (2011) 233–235
doi:10.1016/S0749-0712(11)00020-5
0749-0712/11/$ – see front matter © 2011 Elsevier Inc. All rights reserved.

hand.theclinics.com

Hemophilic (*continued*)
    radiographic features of, 154
    surgical synovectomy and debridement in,
      158–159

I

Implants, linked elbow, and unlinked, compared, 199
Infection, following linked total elbow arthroplasty,
    210
Instability, following linked total elbow arthroplasty,
    211
Interposition arthroplasty, of elbow, **187–197**
    indications for, 188
    rehabilitation following, 195–196
    technique of, 188–195

J

Joint replacement arthroplasty, in hemophilic
    arthropathy, 159–160

L

Linked total elbow arthroplasty. See *Total elbow
    arthroplasty, linked*.
Loosening, aseptic, following linked total elbow
    arthroplasty, 209

M

Medial collateral ligament, reconstruction of, 188, 194

N

Nerves, complications of, following linked total elbow
    arthroplasty, 211
Neuritis, transient median, following osteocapsular
    debridement of elbow, 168
Nonunions, linked total elbow arthroplasty in, 209

O

Ossification, heterotopic, following linked total elbow
    arthroplasty, 211
Osteoarthritis. See also *Arthritis*.
    and posttraumatic arthritis, 200, 202
    linked total elbow arthroplasty in, 209
    primary, and posttraumatic arthritis, of elbow,
      131–137
      of elbow, background and pathogenesis of,
        131
        history taking in, 132–133
        physical examination in, 133
        treatment principles in, 134–136

Osteocapsular debridement, for primary arthritis of
    elbow, **165–170**
    lateral approach for, 166, 167
    medial approach for, 166–167
    patient evaluation in, 165–166
    pitfalls of, 168–169
    posterior approach for, 167–168
    results of, 169
    technique of, 166–168
Outerbridge-Kashiwagi procedure, 134

P

Posttraumatic arthritis, and osteoarthritis, 200, 202
    of elbow, background and pathogenesis of,
      131–132
      history taking in, 132–133
      physical examination in, 133
      treatment principles in, 134–136
Prosthetics, articulation problems, following linked
    total elbow arthroplasty, 211
    fractures of, following linked total elbow
      arthroplasty, 210

R

Radial head arthroplasty, 135
Radiocapitellar joint, hemiarthroplasty of, **229–232**
    case reports of, 229–230
Rheumatoid arthritis, American College of
    Rheumatology classification criteria for, 140
    distraction interposition arthroplasty in, 144–145
    grades of, 141
    linked total elbow arthroplasty in, 208
    of elbow, classification of, 142
      clinical features of, 139–140
      imaging in, 140–141
      postoperative rehabilitation protocols in, 147
      preoperative care in, 142–143
      surgical options in, 143–148
      treatment of, 141–142
    radiographs of patient with, 189
    synovectomy in, 143–144
    total elbow arthroplasty in, 200, 201

S

Synovectomy, in rheumatoid arthritis, 143–144
    surgical, and debridement, in hemophilic
      arthropathy, 158–159
Synoviorthesis, 158

T

Total elbow arthroplasty, 136, 142–143
    axis of rotation of, linked total elbow arthropathy
      and, 207
    complications of, 143–144, 225

contraindications to, 201
convertible, implants for, 221, 222, 223, 224
    rationale for, 220–221
    rehabilitation following, 224–225
    surgical technique for latitude system in,
        221–224
discussion of, 196
in advanced stages of arthritis, 145–147
in elbow nonunion, 201, 203
in rheumatoid arthritis, 200, 201
indications for, 199–201, 215
infection rates in, 143
linked, **199–213**
    aseptic loosening following, 210
    assembly of final components in, 208
    bearing and prosthetic articulation problems
        following, 210–211
    collateral ligament repair and, 208
    complications of, 209–211
    heterotopic ossification following, 211
    humeral preparation for, 206–207
    in acute elbow ankylosis, 209
    in acute elbow fractures, 209
    in acute elbow nonunions, 209
    in osteoarthritis and posttraumatic arthritis,
        209
    in rheumatoid arthritis, 208
    infection following, 210
    instability following, 211
    nerve-related complications following, 211
    prosthetic fractures and periprosthetic
        fractures following, 210
    radial head preparation for, 207
    results of, 208
    TEA axis of rotation and, 207
    trial reduction of implant in, 207–208

    triceps insufficiency following, 211
    triceps reconstruction in, 208
    ulnar preparation for, 207
semiconstrained, 187, 196
surgical approach for, anterior and posterior joint
    capsule, 205
    collateral ligaments and, 205
    osseous structures, 206
    skin and, 205
    triceps insertion and, 205
    ulnar nerve and, 205
surgical technique for, 201–205
    equipment needed for, 204, 205
    general considerations in, 203–204
    patient positioning for, 204
unlinked, and convertible, **215–227**
    biomechanics of, 216, 217
    capitellocondylar, 216
    contraindications to, 215
    Kudo device for, 218
    outcomes of, 147
    prerequisites for, 215
    Pritchard ERS implant for, 216–217
    radial head replacement in, 219–220
    Sorbie-Questor prosthesis for, 218, 219
    Souter-Strathclyde implant for, 218
Triceps insufficiency, following linked total elbow
    arthroplasty, 211

U

Ulnohumeral joint, hemiarthroplasty of, **229–232**
    case reports of, 229–230
Unlinked total elbow arthroplasty. See *Total elbow
    arthroplasty, unlinked*.

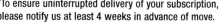

Printed and bound by CPI Group (UK) Ltd, Croydon, CR0 4YY

03/10/2024

01040356-0011